Introduction

You may be someone with high-grade lymphoma. Perhaps someone close to you has this kind of lymphoma. You are not alone: lymphoma is the fifth most common cancer in the UK – more than 14,000 people are diagnosed with it each year, and more than 6,000 of them have high-grade non-Hodgkin lymphoma.

High-grade non-Hodgkin lymphoma covers many different fast-growing lymphomas. These lymphomas need treatment quickly but for most people there is a chance of cure. This booklet will help you to understand more about high-grade lymphoma and what happens during its treatment.

> 'When I was diagnosed with high-grade non-Hodgkin lymphoma, I didn't know what lymphoma was, let alone the types and subtypes. I'm still learning so much.'

Lymphomas are complex, so sometimes we and your doctors and nurses will have to use medical words. To help you understand these, we will explain what they mean when we use them or in the glossary. Words marked like **this** can be found in the glossary.

People often want to know more about their own kind of high-grade lymphoma. Part 5 of this booklet gives more details about many of the common high-grade lymphomas. It tells you how each type differs from other lymphomas.

Because we have covered many different treatments and many high-grade lymphomas, we don't recommend that you read the whole of this booklet from cover to cover. In Parts 4 and 5, we suggest that you read only the sections about your own type of high-grade lymphoma or about treatments that you are going to have. Looking at sections about other lymphomas could be confusing or even misleading.

People with lymphoma and those close to them often tell us it feels like they're on an emotional rollercoaster. It can be hard dealing with the practical problems that can happen during your treatment too.

→ You will find more about the sorts of feelings people often have and some ways you might help yourself or your loved one in Part 6 (see page 113). You will find tips for coping with side effects in the appendix at the end of this booklet.

This booklet is about high-grade non-Hodgkin lymphoma in adults. We have other information about lymphomas in children and booklets specially written for young people with lymphoma.

If you would like to talk to someone about lymphoma or have any questions please ring our Freephone confidential helpline (0808 808 5555), email us on information@lymphomas.org.uk or contact us via Live Chat on our website (www.lymphomas.org.uk). Here you will also find several active forums where you can post messages and share your experiences.

Acknowledgements

This booklet is the fifth edition of a booklet first published in 2006. We would like to thank our Medical Advisory Panel, Lymphoma Nurse Specialists and other expert advisers for their ongoing help in developing our publications. In particular we would like to thank these experts for their help in the 2014 revision of this booklet:

Dr Chris Hatton, Consultant Haematologist, Oxford Radcliffe Hospitals NHS Trust

Frances Penny, Lymphoma Clinical Nurse Specialist, Royal Free London NHS Foundation Trust

Thank you also to all those people affected by lymphoma who have helped us by making suggestions on what to include or by reviewing the revised text.

Finally, thank you to all those who continue to offer support to others affected by lymphoma through our website and forums – some of their words of support and encouragement have been used as quotes in this booklet.

Disclaimer

We make every effort to make sure that the information we give you is accurate but it should not be relied upon to reflect the current state of medical research, which is constantly changing. If you are concerned about your health, you should consult your doctor. The Lymphoma Association cannot accept liability for any loss or damage resulting from any inaccuracy in this information or third party information such as information on websites which we link to.

The information in this booklet can be made available in large print.

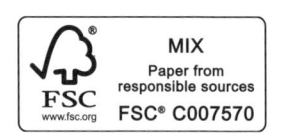

MIX
Paper from responsible sources
FSC® C007570
www.fsc.org

Contents

1 Understanding high-grade non-Hodgkin lymphoma — 9

The lymphatic system — 10
What is lymphoma? — 11
How and why do lymphomas develop? — 12
Symptoms of lymphoma — 13
How are lymphomas classified? — 14
   What does T-cell or B-cell non-Hodgkin lymphoma mean? — 15
   What does 'high-grade' mean? — 16
Key facts — 16

2 Diagnosis and staging — 17

How is lymphoma diagnosed? — 18
   Having a biopsy — 18
Other tests you may need — 19
   Blood tests — 20
   Bone marrow biopsy — 20
   X-rays and scans — 21
   Lumbar puncture — 24
What does the 'stage' mean? — 25
Key facts — 26

3 Treatment overview for high-grade non-Hodgkin lymphoma — 27

About your treatment — 28
Planning treatment — 28
Where will I be treated? — 29
Will my doctor help me to decide about having treatment? — 30
Research and clinical trials — 31

Treatments for high-grade non-Hodgkin lymphoma — 32
Lymphoma treatments in older people — 34

What happens during treatment? — 35
Day-to-day life — 35
Holidays and special events — 37
Sex and contraception — 38

What happens after treatment? — 39
Remission and cure — 39
Follow-up — 40

What happens if high-grade lymphoma comes back? — 41

Key facts — 42

4 More about treatments for high-grade non-Hodgkin lymphoma — 43

Chemotherapy — 44
What is chemotherapy? — 44
How is chemotherapy given? — 44

Side effects of chemotherapy	48
Other treatments sometimes given with chemotherapy	57
CHOP chemotherapy	59
Other chemotherapy regimens	60
Antibody therapy	**60**
What is antibody therapy?	60
How is antibody therapy given?	61
Side effects of antibody therapy	62
Other targeted therapies	**62**
What are targeted therapies?	62
How are targeted therapies given?	65
Side effects of targeted therapies	65
Radiotherapy	**66**
What is radiotherapy?	66
How is radiotherapy given?	66
Side effects of radiotherapy	67
Stem cell transplants	**72**
Key facts	**74**

5 Types of high-grade non-Hodgkin lymphoma — 77

B-cell non-Hodgkin lymphomas	**79**
Diffuse large B-cell lymphoma	79
Burkitt lymphoma	82
Mantle cell lymphoma	86
Primary mediastinal large B-cell lymphoma	89
Primary central nervous system lymphoma (including primary intraocular lymphoma)	90

T-cell non-Hodgkin lymphomas — 94
   Lymphoblastic lymphoma — 94
   Peripheral T-cell lymphoma — 97
   Anaplastic large cell lymphoma — 98
   Angioimmunoblastic T-cell lymphoma — 101
   Enteropathy-associated T-cell lymphoma — 102
   Adult T-cell leukaemia/lymphoma — 104
   Nasal-type NK/T-cell lymphoma — 107

Non-Hodgkin lymphomas associated with immunodeficiency — 109
   Post-transplant lymphoproliferative disorder — 109
   HIV-related lymphoma — 110

6 Looking after yourself — 113

Your feelings — 114

Helping yourself — 117
   Look after your general health and fitness — 117
   Find out about your lymphoma — 118

When someone close to you has lymphoma — 118

Key facts — 120

Help and support — 121

Glossary — 123

Useful organisations — 127

Selected references — 129

**Appendix:
Tips for coping with treatment side effects** — 130

Understanding high-grade non-Hodgkin lymphoma

The lymphatic system

What is lymphoma?

How and why do lymphomas develop?

Symptoms of lymphoma

How are lymphomas classified?

High-grade non-Hodgkin lymphoma

1 The lymphatic system

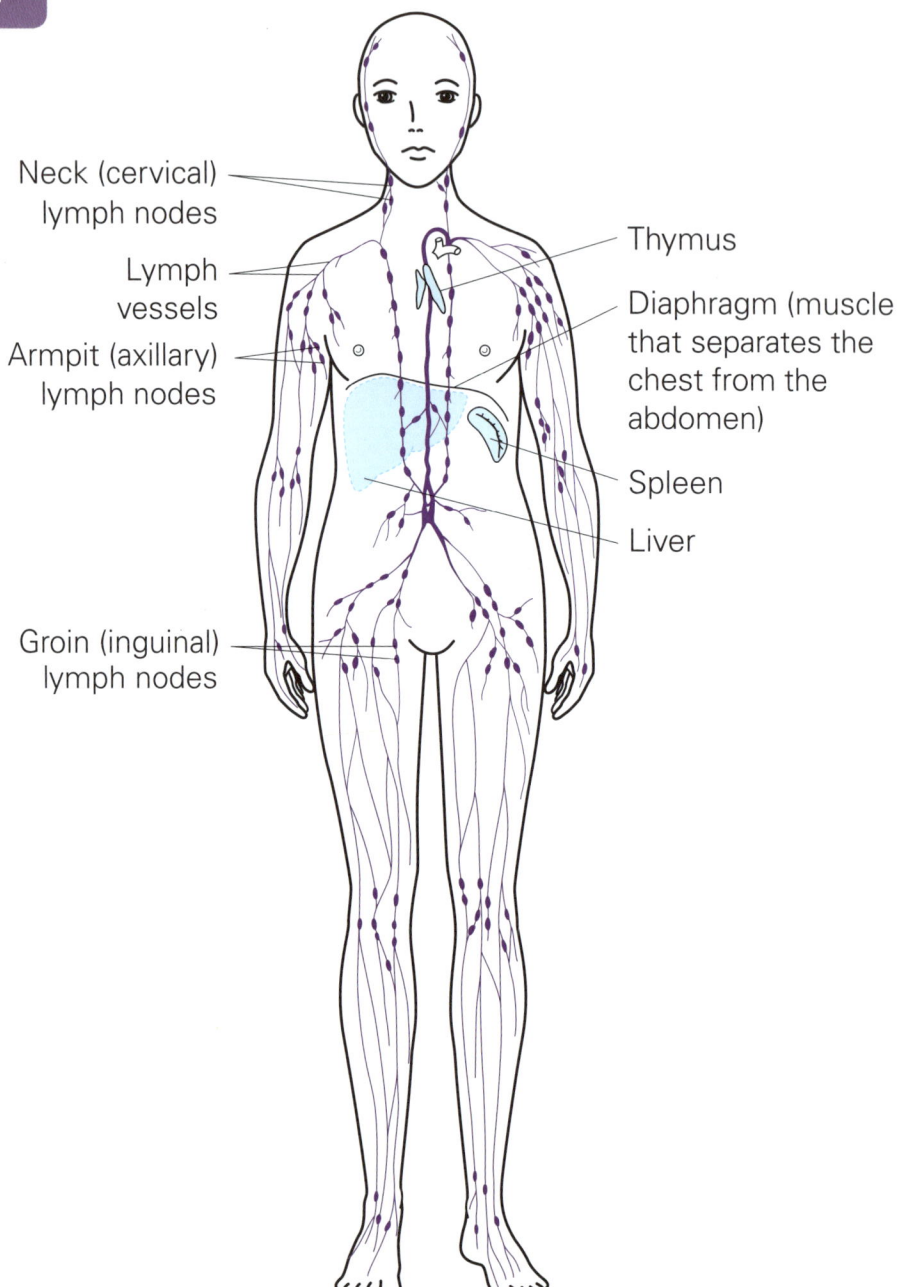

- Neck (cervical) lymph nodes
- Lymph vessels
- Armpit (axillary) lymph nodes
- Thymus
- Diaphragm (muscle that separates the chest from the abdomen)
- Spleen
- Liver
- Groin (inguinal) lymph nodes

Our lymphatic system is made up of a complex network of tubes (known as lymph vessels), glands (known as **lymph nodes**) and other organs such as the **spleen**. We have lymph nodes and lymph vessels throughout our bodies. Some groups of lymph nodes may be easily felt, for example under the arms, in the neck and in the groin; others are deeper inside us and can only be seen on scans.

The lymphatic system is part of the body's natural defence against infection – the **immune system**. The lymph nodes are an important part of this defence, acting as a sieve in the lymphatic system. They are a home to large numbers of **lymphocytes** (a type of **white blood cell** that helps our bodies to fight infection).

> If you would like to know more about the lymphatic and immune systems please ring our helpline (0808 808 5555), email us on information@lymphomas.org.uk or see our website (www.lymphomas.org.uk).

What is lymphoma?

Lymphomas are cancers of the lymphatic system. They occur when some of the lymphocytes become cancerous.

Lymphoma is not just one illness. There are many different kinds but they all start with a cancerous lymphocyte.

Lymphoma was first described in the 19th century by Dr Thomas Hodgkin. One kind of lymphoma known as Hodgkin lymphoma (or Hodgkin's disease) is named after him; all other kinds are known as non-Hodgkin lymphoma.

Each year more than 12,000 people are diagnosed with non-Hodgkin lymphoma in the UK. It can occur at any age, including in children, but it becomes steadily more common in people aged 50 and over.

> 'To say the diagnosis was a shock is an understatement. I was always very active and loved keeping on the move.'

How and why do lymphomas develop?

Our lymphocytes are always dividing to make new lymphocytes. When fighting an infection, lots of new lymphocytes are made very quickly. Only those that target the infection we have at the time are useful to the immune system. Any lymphocytes that do not target that infection will die, meaning it is only the useful lymphocytes that survive. All of this usually happens in a carefully controlled way.

Lymphomas can occur when there is a breakdown in the control of this system. Instead of dying in the normal way, untargeted 'rogue' lymphocytes start to divide in an uncontrolled way. The rogue lymphocytes collect together to form a lump, most commonly in a **lymph node**. This is a lymphoma.

The rogue lymphocytes can also collect in other parts of the body to form lymphoma. These areas, such as the **spleen**, liver, gut, skin and **bone marrow**, are known as **extranodal** sites.

For most lymphomas, the exact trigger that causes the changes and makes the lymphocytes become cancerous is still unknown. Despite this, it is important that you know:
- You have not done anything to yourself to cause lymphoma.
- You did not inherit it from your parents.
- You didn't catch it and you can't pass it on to others.

Although anyone can develop a lymphoma, some people are more at risk of lymphoma. This may be because their immune system does not work well (known as **immunodeficiency**). It can occur in people who have **HIV** infection or people who have had an organ transplant, for example. There is a section of this booklet about lymphomas associated with immunodeficiency (see pages 109–112).

Some kinds of lymphoma are known to be linked with certain **viruses**. We have highlighted this in the detailed information about those lymphomas.

Symptoms of lymphoma

People with lymphoma can have many different **symptoms**. Some of the symptoms are common to many cancers. For instance, the lymphoma cells take up energy and nutrients that are needed by healthy cells, so people often feel very tired.

The commonest symptom of lymphoma is:
- a painless lump or swelling, often in the neck, armpit or groin. This is a swollen **lymph node**.

Other possible symptoms include:
- weight loss for no obvious reason ⎤
- drenching sweats, especially at night ⎬ these are known as **B symptoms**
- fever and flu-like symptoms that don't go away ⎦
- rash or itching.

Sometimes people can have lymphoma in other parts of the body, including the stomach, lungs, skin or brain. In this case there may not be any lymph nodes or other lumps to feel. Symptoms can vary, depending on where the lymphoma is. For example, lymphoma can cause:
- abdominal pain
- diarrhoea or change in bowel habit
- jaundice
- a persistent cough or breathlessness.

> 'My husband has been diagnosed with diffuse large B-cell lymphoma – it's been a huge shock as he hasn't been ill, maybe a bit tired but he just had a lump on his neck.'

There is no one symptom that is unique to lymphoma, but a mixture of these symptoms is typical. If the lymphoma isn't treated, more symptoms will occur and the symptoms will get worse over time.

How are lymphomas classified?

There are different kinds of lymphocyte, any of which can become cancerous, so there are also many different types of lymphoma.

Lymphomas are classified (or divided and sorted) in three broad ways:
- Hodgkin lymphoma or non-Hodgkin lymphoma
- T-cell or B-cell non-Hodgkin lymphoma
- high-grade or low-grade non-Hodgkin lymphoma.

Doctors will classify your lymphoma by looking in detail at the cells. They will want to know what the cells look like under the microscope and what **proteins** they have on their surface. Other specialised tests may also be needed, for example tests to find out about any changes affecting the genes within the lymphoma cells.

The classification of your lymphoma is very important. It will give your doctor vital information about your illness and tell them:
- what kind of lymphocyte has become cancerous
- whether the lymphoma is growing quickly or slowly
- how the lymphoma may behave, for example what parts of your body are likely to be affected
- what kind of treatment you will need – certain types of lymphoma need different treatments from others.

What does T-cell or B-cell non-Hodgkin lymphoma mean?

Lymphomas happen when a **lymphocyte** divides in an uncontrolled way because it has become cancerous. Lymphocytes are either B lymphocytes (often known as **B cells**) or T lymphocytes (**T cells**).

B cells and T cells mature in different parts of the body: B cells in the bone marrow; T cells in the thymus (a gland found in the chest). Both cells help protect the body from infection and illness but do so in slightly different ways.

A cancerous B cell can become a B-cell lymphoma; a cancerous T cell can become a T-cell lymphoma. B-cell lymphomas are much more common than T-cell lymphomas in the UK.

What does 'high-grade' mean?
Non-Hodgkin lymphomas are described as either high grade or low grade. 'High grade' means the cells are dividing quickly, so this is a fast-growing kind of lymphoma. You may also hear the word 'aggressive' used to describe high-grade lymphoma. This may sound alarming but actually many high-grade non-Hodgkin lymphomas have a better chance of being cured than low-grade or slow-growing non-Hodgkin lymphomas.

Key facts

Lymphomas are cancers of the lymphatic system. They develop when some of the lymphocytes become cancerous and start to grow out of control. There are many different types of lymphoma.

Lymphomas may cause very few symptoms. The commonest symptom is a painless lump – a swollen lymph node. Other symptoms include weight loss, night sweats and tiredness.

Lymphomas are either Hodgkin lymphoma (Hodgkin's disease) or non-Hodgkin lymphoma. Non-Hodgkin lymphomas can be fast growing (high grade) or slow growing (low grade).

They may develop from B cells or T cells. B-cell lymphomas are more common than T-cell lymphomas.

Diagnosis and staging

2

How is lymphoma diagnosed?

Other tests you may need

What does the 'stage' mean?

How is lymphoma diagnosed?

The word **diagnosis** simply means finding out what is wrong. In most cases, it is not possible for a GP to confirm whether or not you have lymphoma – not even from a blood test. Your GP will send you to a doctor at a hospital for further tests. These will almost certainly include a **biopsy**.

There are many different types of lymphoma and making an accurate diagnosis is vital.

Having a biopsy
For most people a biopsy is the only way to tell whether or not a lump is lymphoma. It is a test that removes some of your cells so they can be looked at under a microscope.

The method used to take your biopsy will depend on where your swollen **lymph nodes** are found and what the doctors in your hospital prefer to do. **Note:** if you are taking medicines to thin your blood, you may be asked to stop these for a while before having your biopsy.

If you have a node that can easily be felt, a surgeon may remove either all or part of it (an 'excision biopsy'). Sometimes a **radiologist** may take a small sample of the lymph node (a 'core biopsy') instead.

If your swollen nodes are all deep inside you, a surgeon may need to remove either part or all of a node using laparoscopic (key-hole) surgery. Instead of this, a radiologist may be able to take a core biopsy. They will usually scan you at the same time to make sure they test the right area.

If you have an excision biopsy or laparoscopic surgery, you will need to have a general **anaesthetic**. Most people need to stay in hospital at least for a night after a laparoscopic biopsy. This may also be the case after an excision biopsy. For a core biopsy, you will probably only need a local anaesthetic and may be able to go home the same day.

Sometimes the biopsy will be taken from other areas that may be affected, such as the **bone marrow** (see page 20).

The biopsy will be looked at under the microscope by an expert lymphoma **pathologist**.

If needed, the pathologist will arrange further tests on the biopsy to decide exactly what type of lymphoma you have. This is why it is important that the biopsy taken is big enough for all the tests to be done – if there isn't enough tissue sometimes a second biopsy is needed.

Other tests you may need

Your doctors may want you to have other tests as well as your biopsy. This section is about some of the common tests for lymphoma, but don't worry if you don't have all of these tests. Sometimes only a few of them are needed to find out about your lymphoma.

For most of these tests you can be an outpatient, meaning you won't have to stay in hospital overnight. It may take a couple of weeks for all the results to be available.

It is normal for you to feel anxious while waiting for these tests and the results. It's very important though that your doctors have all the information they need about your lymphoma. This will help them choose the most suitable treatment for you.

Blood tests

You will have blood samples taken before you start treatment and regularly during treatment. Blood tests are done for many reasons:
- to check for **anaemia** or other low blood cell counts
- to check that your kidneys and liver are working well
- to give your doctors an idea of how your lymphoma may behave
- to look for infections such as hepatitis or **HIV**, which may also need treatment or could flare up with lymphoma treatments.

Bone marrow biopsy

The **bone marrow** is the spongy, jelly-like middle part of some of our bones and it is where blood cells are made. Your doctors may want you to have a bone marrow biopsy to see if there are any lymphoma cells there. They may also call this test a bone marrow 'aspirate' or bone marrow 'trephine'.

If you are taking medicines to thin your blood, you may be asked to stop these beforehand. The whole test takes around 15–20 minutes.

A sample of bone marrow is usually taken from your hip bone using a special biopsy needle. The skin and area over the bone is first numbed with a local **anaesthetic**. Despite this, taking the sample can still sometimes be

Diagnosis and staging

painful, although it is usually done very quickly. Sedatives or Entonox® (gas and air) can help some people, but you'll need to talk to your doctor as they aren't always advisable.

X-rays and scans

X-rays
X-rays can be used to look at various parts of your body. For example, a chest X-ray may be used to see if there are any swollen **lymph nodes** in your chest. X-rays are painless and shouldn't take longer than a few minutes.

CT scans
Computed tomography (CT) scans use a series of X-rays to form pictures of your body in cross-section, like 'slices' through your body.

The test involves lying on a padded table that moves your body into a doughnut-shaped camera. The space is quite open so you shouldn't feel 'hemmed in' or claustrophobic. As the table moves, the camera takes pictures of the different layers of your body.

You might be given a special dye (a contrast agent) to drink or as an injection before the scan. This makes it easier to see some of your internal organs. The scan is painless and usually takes only a few minutes. You will be asked to lie quite still while the pictures are being taken. You might also be asked to hold your breath for up to 20 seconds at some stage during the scan.

Talk to the staff in the department if you are worried about any aspect of having your CT scan done.

MRI scans

Magnetic resonance imaging (MRI) scans are similar to CT scans, except they make pictures of you using strong magnets and radio waves instead of X-rays. The pictures are slightly different and are particularly good for looking at certain tissues such as the brain.

You'll be asked to lie on a padded table that moves you into a cylinder (tube). The cylinder measures radio waves as they pass through your body. The test is painless but can take up to an hour. If you would find it uncomfortable to lie still for this long, you might need to take painkillers beforehand, but ask your doctor about this.

The scanner can be very noisy and, as you are in a small space, you may feel claustrophobic (hemmed in). You'll be asked to take off any metal jewellery and clothing with metal parts that could be magnetic. The staff will also ask if you have any metal implants, such as a hip replacement or a pacemaker.

Let the staff in the department know if you are worried about any aspect of having an MRI scan done.

PET scans

Positron-emission tomography (PET) scans can help doctors work out which cells in your body are cancerous and which are not. They use a radioactive sugar to show up the most active cells in the body, and lymphoma cells are usually very active.

A CT scan is often done at the same time and this is called a 'PET/CT scan'. It can give a clearer picture of exactly which areas are cancerous.

Diagnosis and staging

Having the scan is painless and the whole process usually takes about 2–3 hours.

It is very like having a CT scan but it is important to carefully follow any advice you are given about what to do before and after your scan. If you have diabetes, you'll be given special instructions to help you keep your sugar levels stable.

If you have any concerns about having a PET scan, talk to the staff in the department – they understand that this scan is something new for most people.

PET/CT scans are now done for many people with high-grade non-Hodgkin lymphoma. They are a good way to check what parts of the body the lymphoma is affecting. This can be important when your doctors decide which treatment you should have. They may also be done later, to check how well your treatment has worked and whether you need any more treatment.

Doctors are continuing to learn how best to use these scans. Clinical trials are testing whether having a scan just a month or two into treatment may be useful. This might show how the lymphoma is responding early on during treatment.

If the doctors know that there is a good response, they could possibly recommend giving less treatment. If the PET scan still shows active lymphoma, they might suggest trying a different treatment, which could perhaps work better.

Lumbar puncture

Your brain and spinal cord are cushioned by a fluid called the cerebrospinal fluid (CSF). Lymphoma cells can be found in the CSF in some kinds of high-grade lymphoma. Your doctor may want to look at some of this fluid with a microscope to see if any lymphoma cells are present. If they do, you will need to have a lumbar puncture (spinal tap).

You can eat and drink as normal before having a lumbar puncture. But if you are taking medicines to thin your blood, you may be asked to stop these beforehand.

Typically, while you are having the test, you will be asked to lie on your side with your knees pulled up towards your chest. A doctor will pass a special needle between the bones of your spine in the small of your back. You will have an injection of local **anaesthetic** first to numb the area. A small amount of CSF (about 3–4 teaspoons) will be drained off and sent to the laboratory for testing.

You shouldn't find this test painful, except that the local anaesthetic can sting. You will need to keep very still during the test and to stay lying down afterwards, possibly for a few hours.

Please contact us if you would like to talk to someone about your tests or if you would like further information. You can ring our Freephone helpline on 0808 808 5555, email us on information@lymphomas.org.uk or contact us via Live Chat on our website (www.lymphomas.org.uk).

Diagnosis and staging

What does the 'stage' mean?

Once all the test results are ready, your doctor will be able to tell which parts of your body are affected by your lymphoma. This is called the 'stage' of your lymphoma. It will be important in planning your treatment. These are the different stages used for most high-grade lymphomas.

Stage I	One group of **lymph nodes** affected
Stage II	Two or more groups of lymph nodes affected on one side of the **diaphragm**
Stage III	Lymph nodes affected on both sides of the **diaphragm**
Stage IV	Lymphoma can be found either in the **bone marrow** or in organs that are not part of the lymphatic system

Letters can be added to the stage too. 'B' would mean you have B symptoms (weight loss, night sweats or fevers); 'A' would mean you have none of these.

Other letters are added less often. A letter 'E' would mean you have **extranodal** lymphoma (lymphoma outside your lymphatic system). A letter 'X' would mean you have 'bulky disease'. This means you have a group of lymph nodes that are very large and this area may need extra treatment.

Stage I lymphomas, and some stage II lymphomas, are referred to as **early-stage** (localised) lymphoma. Some stage II lymphomas – those with large lumps or causing symptoms – are grouped with the stage III and IV lymphomas. These are referred to as **advanced-stage** lymphoma. This may sound alarming but there are good treatments available for lymphoma at all disease stages. High-grade lymphoma is not like some other cancers where advanced stage may mean the cancer cannot be cured or there are few treatments available.

If you are not sure whether your lymphoma is early stage or advanced stage, we suggest you check with your doctor – the treatments for these stages can be quite different.

Key facts

Lymphoma is normally diagnosed by a biopsy. This means that cells are removed to be looked at under the microscope.

Usually a swollen lymph node is sampled – either by removing all or part of it, or by taking a smaller 'core' biopsy. A number of special tests will be done on the sample to decide what type of lymphoma you have.

You will need to have other tests, such as blood tests, a bone marrow biopsy and scans.

The results allow your doctors to work out the stage of your lymphoma. This information is important in planning the right treatment for you.

Treatment overview for high-grade non-Hodgkin lymphoma

3

About your treatment

Treatments for high-grade non-Hodgkin lymphoma

What happens during treatment?

What happens after treatment?

What happens if high-grade lymphoma comes back?

About your treatment

Planning treatment
Once your doctors have the results of all the tests, they will be able to plan your treatment. Your doctors are part of a team known as a multidisciplinary team (MDT). The team includes other experts who look after people with lymphoma too. They will meet to check all your test results and think about the most suitable treatment for you.

This will depend on:
- the exact type of lymphoma you have
- the stage of your lymphoma.

Other points they will think about include:
- your thoughts on treatment and what is important to you
- your general health and usual level of fitness
- any other illnesses you have and how these affect you
- the size of your lumps
- your blood test results.

Finishing the tests and planning your treatment can take a couple of weeks. This might seem a long time, but the information being collected is very important. Your doctor needs to know as much as possible about you and your lymphoma before choosing the best treatment for you.

You will probably feel worried when you are waiting to find out more or waiting to start your treatment – this is only natural. You may find it helps to talk about this to someone, maybe a specialist nurse or your GP.

Where will I be treated?

People with lymphoma can be treated at local hospitals or at larger hospitals that have a specialist cancer centre. Sometimes the treatment is shared between the two.

Your GP, or the doctor who finds out that you have lymphoma, will send you to the nearest hospital with a doctor who is an expert in treating lymphoma. You may see either a **haematologist** (a doctor who specialises in treating blood problems) or an **oncologist** (a doctor who specialises in treating cancer).

If you have a rare type of lymphoma you may be referred to a specialist cancer centre. The doctors there are likely to have seen more people with your type of lymphoma. They may also be running a clinical trial that you could enter if you wanted. The doctor at your local hospital might still treat you nearer home with guidance from the cancer centre.

Your doctor will not mind if you want to ask questions about your hospital and how they plan to give you the care you need.

Other questions that might be important to ask are:
- Will your doctor meet regularly with other lymphoma experts at an MDT meeting?
- Does the hospital have a clinical nurse specialist or other specialist cancer nurse?
- Does the hospital take part in clinical trials?
- What other experts are there to help if you need them? For example, will you be able to see a dietitian or a counsellor if you need to?

Will my doctor help me to decide about having treatment?

For many people with high-grade lymphoma, the decision to go ahead with treatment is simple. Generally, these will be people who are quite fit and have a good chance of cure with the standard treatment. They will usually begin treatment quite quickly, as treatment also normally helps to ease any symptoms the lymphoma is causing.

For other people, the decision to go ahead with treatment may be harder. Perhaps the treatment is less likely to cure their lymphoma. They may be at more risk of side effects with the treatment. Sometimes, it can be hard to weigh up all the benefits and the risks, especially if there is more than one possible treatment – for example, a strong treatment and another that is more gentle.

> 'It is worrying at the start as there is so much unknown and for most of us it is a world we never imagined we would be in.'

Your doctor will help you decide what treatment to have. It is important you are happy that whatever decision you make is the right one for you. Talk to your doctor, clinical nurse specialist, and family and friends who are supporting you if you are finding it hard to make a decision. Make sure you understand the treatment being recommended for you and any choices you have. Ask as many questions as you need to help you with your decision.

Many people find it helps to take a relative or friend along to their hospital appointments. Your companion may remember things that are said that you don't recall. They may remind you of other questions that they know you wanted to ask. Your doctor won't mind. In fact most doctors will encourage their patients to bring someone along. You may want to take a notebook and pen with you too in case you want to write anything down.

> For more ideas about what to ask your medical team please ring our helpline (0808 808 5555) or see our website (www.lymphomas.org.uk).

Research and clinical trials

You may be asked if you would like to take part in a clinical trial. These are scientific studies that test medical treatments.

Some trials are designed to test new treatments that haven't yet been tried in a particular type of lymphoma. Others are looking to improve on the current treatments, perhaps by changing one of the drugs or adding in something new. Clinical trials are very important in improving the future treatment of people with lymphoma.

Each clinical trial is usually for people with just one type of lymphoma, or sometimes a few similar types. For some trials, only people in a certain age group will be allowed to take part. Having other illnesses may also stop some people going into a trial, so they are not suitable for everyone.

Not all hospitals take part in clinical trials and some trials will be run in only a few centres. It is important to ask about clinical trials that may be suitable for you, especially if you have a rare type of lymphoma. Your doctor may be able to refer you to another centre if you would like treatment in a clinical trial.

Clinical trials are entirely voluntary. You do not have to take part in a trial if you do not wish to. You can always opt to have the standard treatment if you prefer. It is important you understand fully what is involved before you agree to take part in a trial – you will be given written information. If you change your mind later on, you are free to withdraw from the trial at any time.

If you do take part in a trial, you will be carefully watched or may have more tests. Apart from this, however, you may not get any direct benefit – no one can say which treatment is better until the trial is finished. The one certain fact is that you will be helping other people to have the best possible treatment for lymphoma in the future.

> We produce a booklet on clinical trials. Please ring our helpline (0808 808 5555) or see our website (www.lymphomas.org.uk) if you would like a copy.

Treatments for high-grade non-Hodgkin lymphoma

Which treatment, or treatments, you will have depends mainly on the type of non-Hodgkin lymphoma you have (B-cell or T-cell lymphoma) and its stage. It may not be possible to give the same treatments if you are older or less fit, and we will explain the reasons for this (see pages 34–35).

Treatment overview for high-grade non-Hodgkin lymphoma

If you are not sure what type of lymphoma you have or its stage, you may want to check with your doctor or clinical nurse specialist. Reading about treatments that you aren't likely to have may be confusing or worrying.

Almost everybody who has a high-grade lymphoma will be offered treatment with chemotherapy. The **regimen** (combination of drugs) most often used is called 'CHOP' (described in more detail on page 59). You will be able to see in Part 5 if other regimens are commonly used to treat your type of high-grade lymphoma.

Chemotherapy is normally repeated every few weeks, with the whole treatment often taking several months. Most people with high-grade lymphoma can have their chemotherapy in a day treatment unit. Some types of high-grade lymphoma are, however, better treated with stronger regimens that can only be given to people who are inpatients.

For people with a B-cell lymphoma, an **antibody** is usually given with the chemotherapy. Most often, the antibody used is rituximab (described in more detail on pages 61–62). A letter 'R' is added to the name when rituximab is part of the regimen, for example R-CHOP.

Some people with high-grade lymphoma will be treated with radiotherapy as well as chemotherapy. Radiotherapy on its own is used only rarely for people with high-grade lymphoma.

Early-stage lymphoma is often treated with a short course of chemotherapy followed by radiotherapy. Advanced-stage lymphoma is treated with longer courses of chemotherapy. After this, radiotherapy usually isn't needed, except for people who had 'bulky disease' (areas with very large **lymph nodes** before treatment).

Lymphoma treatments in older people

More than half of people diagnosed with non-Hodgkin lymphoma are over 65. Treatments for non-Hodgkin lymphoma sometimes have to be adjusted in older people to make them safer. Doctors will not decide your treatment based on your age, but will think very carefully about any other health problems you have. Such problems often become more common as people get older.

Your doctors will need to be sure that the treatment they are recommending is safe for you. For example, if your heart isn't working well, they may avoid giving you certain drugs that could make it worse.

Sometimes people who are older can be more troubled by side effects and may take longer to recover from them. Your doctors may adjust your treatment to lower the chances of you getting side effects.

If you are older or less fit, your treatment will be carefully planned just for you. It will depend in particular on how well your heart, lungs and kidneys are working. Your doctors may arrange for you to have special tests, such as an echocardiogram (often just called an 'echo') or lung function tests, before you start any treatment. Talk to your team about what is happening and why.

Your doctors will want to give you as much treatment for your lymphoma as they feel is safe. They will balance this against the risks of making you more ill with the treatment and its likely complications. This might mean that your treatment has to be slightly different from the treatments we describe for younger people.

There are a number of clinical trials now looking at the best ways to treat people with lymphoma who are older or less fit. Some of these involve changing treatment regimens to make them easier to cope with. Others are looking at adding newer drugs to current chemotherapy, which may help the treatments work better.

Don't be afraid to ask your doctor about your treatment and why they feel it is the best treatment for you. Your doctor will also be able to tell you whether there are any suitable clinical trials for you to enter.

What happens during treatment?

Day-to-day life
It is hard to predict exactly how you will feel during your treatment and how it will affect your day-to-day life. If you have had lots of symptoms from your lymphoma, you may feel much better once you start treatment. Some people have few side effects from their treatment and are able to carry on almost as normal; others will have side effects that mean they need to make changes, at least for a while.

> 'It is a rollercoaster ride, with highs and lows, good days and bad. Focus on the good days and try to enjoy them.'

➡️ More information on possible side effects is given on pages 48–57 for chemotherapy, page 62 for antibody therapy and pages 67–72 for radiotherapy.

Working

If you normally work, you should let your employers know what is happening – most will be sympathetic and flexible, and you have a number of rights in law.

At the very least, you are going to need to take time off work for hospital appointments. In practice, most people take a lot more time off or need to work fewer hours or change the work they are doing. Your hospital team will be able to offer you more advice depending on your treatment and the sort of work you do.

If you are unable to work, you will probably be entitled to sick pay. This will not be the case if you are self-employed. In this case you will need to try to plan how you will manage your work and finances.

If you are unemployed, you should advise your local Department for Work and Pensions (DWP) office of your illness as your benefit payments will probably change.

Ask at your hospital as they may have a specialist benefits/welfare adviser that you could see.

📞 Please ring our helpline if you would like to talk about work and benefits (0808 808 5555). Macmillan Cancer Support produce detailed information about work and cancer – see page 128 for their contact details.

Hobbies and socialising

It is important that, while being treated for lymphoma, you allow yourself time to do things you enjoy. When you feel well enough you should try to continue as much as possible with your hobbies – do check with your hospital team if your usual hobbies are adventurous, very active, or in any way dangerous.

You will also probably feel better if you can keep up your social life as far as possible. Seeing a few friends, getting out or having a change of scenery can help to make you feel more 'normal'. Do be aware though that there may be times when you should avoid crowds because of the risk of infection – your hospital team will be able to give you more advice about this.

> 'I was determined to lead as normal a life as possible during the three weeks between rounds of chemo. I went out with my friends, drove to the supermarket and went out for walks.'

Holidays and special events

For most people having treatment for high-grade lymphoma, a holiday, especially outside the UK, may not be the best idea. It may though be possible to make small changes to your planned treatment so that you can be away from home for a while. Do tell your hospital team in plenty of time if you have any special events or plans, so that they can offer you the best advice.

Even if you are thinking about a holiday when you have finished treatment, do talk about this with your team. You might need to think about where you travel to, your accommodation and whether you will need any vaccinations. Finding travel insurance at a reasonable price can also be a problem, so it is important to think ahead.

> For more information about all aspects of travel and holidays please ring our helpline (0808 808 5555) or see our website (www.lymphomas.org.uk).

Sex and contraception

There is no reason why you should not have sex during treatment if you feel like it, but you should continue to use contraceptives during treatment. This is because treatments may damage sperm or eggs and could be harmful to a developing baby. Also, if a woman is pregnant it can make it harder to treat the lymphoma.

Advice varies but doctors will often give this advice to people having chemotherapy:
- Women with lymphoma should not become pregnant during their treatment and for some time afterwards (some doctors recommend 2 years).
  Note: oral contraceptive tablets may not work as well while you are on treatment, so talk to your doctor or nurse about this.
- Men with lymphoma should avoid making their partner pregnant while they are having chemotherapy and for at least 3 months afterwards (some doctors recommend longer).

If this is an issue for you, do talk about it with your hospital team. They will then be able to give you specific advice as your circumstances could be different.

→ You will find more information about the effects of treatment on fertility on pages 55–56.

Traces of chemotherapy can stay in the body for up to 5 days after treatment. Condoms should be used during this time and you should avoid oral sex and open-mouth kissing where saliva is exchanged, as body fluids may contain traces of chemotherapy.

For more information about sexuality and lymphoma please ring our helpline (0808 808 5555) or see our website (www.lymphomas.org.uk).

What happens after treatment?

Remission and cure

Remission means that the lymphoma has been controlled. There are different degrees of remission. A **complete remission** is where no lymphoma can be seen on the scans after treatment. A **partial remission** is where the lymphoma has shrunk by at least a half.

Treatments for high-grade lymphoma are usually aimed at giving you a long-term complete remission, which hopefully will become a cure.

You may find that your doctor prefers to say 'you are in remission' rather than 'you are cured'. This is because they cannot say for certain whether or not your lymphoma will come back. But the longer you have been in remission, the less likely it is that your lymphoma will come back (**relapse**).

A small number of people with high-grade lymphoma will not respond well to treatment. Lymphoma that does not go into remission after treatment is known as **refractory** lymphoma. It is usually treated in the same way as relapsed high-grade lymphoma.

Follow-up

Once your treatment has finished, you will still see your hospital team regularly. These follow-up appointments are to see how you are feeling, to check on your recovery from treatment and to make sure there are no signs of the lymphoma coming back.

You will have a brief physical examination and you may have more blood tests. Unless your doctors think you could be relapsing, you probably won't have scans or X-rays. This is because they are usually not needed and could increase your risk of later side effects.

People who have had high-grade lymphoma will usually be followed for anything up to 5 years after the end of their treatment. Your appointments will probably be around once every 3 months for the first few years. If you stay well, they will be spread out to once every 6–12 months.

If you are worried about your health at any time, you don't have to wait for your next appointment. You should get in touch with your GP or hospital team to talk about your concerns. They might arrange an early clinic appointment for you. Make sure you keep the contact details for your hospital team even after you have finished treatment.

Most people worry about their follow-up appointments. You might not want to go back to the hospital, but these appointments are an important part of your care. They give you a chance to talk about anything that might be on your mind. It can help to write these things down when you think of them and take a list of questions with you.

What happens if high-grade lymphoma comes back?

In some people, high-grade lymphoma will relapse (come back after treatment) and in a smaller number it will be **refractory** (not respond well to the first treatment).

Relapse is most likely to happen within 2 years of the end of your first treatment.

If your lymphoma comes back, your doctor will want to repeat some of the tests you had at the start.

You may be able to have further treatment for your lymphoma. This treatment will depend on:
- how fit you are when you relapse
- the type of treatment you had before and how you responded to that treatment
- how well you coped with the treatment
- how quickly your lymphoma has come back.

Often a different chemotherapy **regimen** can be offered. For some people, a stem cell transplant may be possible too. In some lymphomas, newer drugs are becoming available or are being tested in clinical trials. You may like to ask your doctor if there is a suitable trial for you.

Key facts

Your treatment will be planned just for you so may not be the same as someone else's. You may be asked if you wish to take part in a clinical trial.

Most people with high-grade lymphoma will be treated with chemotherapy. The regimen used most often is called CHOP.

People with high-grade B-cell lymphoma will usually be treated with the antibody rituximab too.

People with early-stage high-grade lymphoma are often treated with a short course of chemotherapy followed by radiotherapy.

Radiotherapy is also used to treat people with advanced-stage high-grade lymphoma if they have an area with very large lymph nodes.

You will continue to see your hospital team for a few years after your treatment.

Relapsed non-Hodgkin lymphoma can be treated again. In people who are fit enough, a stem cell transplant may be possible. There are also many new drugs now being tested in clinical trials.

More about treatments for high-grade non-Hodgkin lymphoma

4

- **Chemotherapy**
- **Antibody therapy**
- **Other targeted therapies**
- **Radiotherapy**
- **Stem cell transplants**

Chemotherapy

What is chemotherapy?
The word 'chemotherapy' means treatment with drugs. Drugs for cancer are called 'cytotoxic' because they kill cells: 'cyto' means cell, and 'toxic' means poisonous.

Chemotherapy works by stopping the cancer cells dividing. Different chemotherapy drugs do this in slightly different ways. Chemotherapy for lymphoma usually involves giving more than one kind of drug. This increases the chances of killing as many cancer cells as possible.

Chemotherapy works particularly well on cells that are dividing quickly and less well on cells that are dormant (resting). To target as many cells as possible, chemotherapy is generally given as repeated blocks of treatment (often called **cycles**). With each treatment cycle, more cells are destroyed and the lymphoma gradually shrinks.

Each cycle also has a rest period when no chemotherapy is given. This is because normal cells, such as those in the **bone marrow** and the lining of the mouth and bowel, are also damaged by chemotherapy. The rest period allows the healthy normal cells time to recover. You may still have other medicines during this time though, for example to protect you from side effects.

How is chemotherapy given?
Chemotherapy for high-grade lymphoma is very often given as an outpatient treatment. This means you will visit hospital on the day of treatment but go home afterwards. Some chemotherapy **regimens** take longer

to give, so a stay in hospital is usually needed. Your doctor will let you know if they are recommending this kind of treatment for you.

You will probably have a number of cycles of chemotherapy (usually six to eight), each taking a few weeks. The exact timetable for your treatment will depend on what kind of chemotherapy you are having. Your hospital team will give you specific information about your treatment and what to expect.

Whatever treatment you are having, you may need to stay in hospital if you get severe side effects, for instance very low blood cell counts or an infection.

→ You will find more information about the most common side effects of chemotherapy on pages 48–57.

Chemotherapy for high-grade lymphoma can be given in a number of different ways:
- intravenously, meaning through a thin tube into a vein (the most common way)
- orally, meaning by mouth in tablet or capsule form
- intrathecally, meaning into the fluid that surrounds your brain and spinal cord (less commonly needed).

Intravenous chemotherapy
Intravenous drugs for high-grade lymphoma are typically given through a cannula (a small plastic tube that goes into a vein, usually on the back of your hand or in your lower arm). Once the drugs have been given, the cannula is taken out. A new one is put in each time.

Some intravenous drugs are given as a 'bolus'. The drug is 'pushed' through the cannula using a syringe, usually over a few minutes. Intravenous chemotherapy can sometimes make your arm sting. Tell the nurse if you feel any discomfort.

Other intravenous drugs are given as a drip (an infusion). The drug is put into a bag of fluid, which then drips through the cannula over many minutes (or sometimes hours). A pump may be used to make sure the drip goes in over the correct time. The drip and the pump are often hung on a stand with wheels, so you can walk around.

People with certain high-grade lymphomas may need to have chemotherapy that is spread over many hours or even days. They will need to be an inpatient for this treatment.

Often this kind of chemotherapy regimen is given through a more permanent intravenous tube (or 'line') instead of through a cannula. This makes it easier and safer to give the drugs that are needed. Sometimes lines are also used for people having problems with cannulas for outpatient chemotherapy.

There are two kinds of line: a PICC line (peripherally inserted central catheter) and a tunnelled central line. A **PICC line** usually goes in through a vein in the arm at the level of the elbow. It's held in place by tape or a dressing. A **tunnelled central line** is usually positioned on the upper chest. Part of the line runs in a tunnel under the skin, which reduces the risk of infection. You may hear these called Hickman® or Groshong® lines.

Such lines can often stay in place for all the cycles of treatment. They must be kept covered and need a bit of extra care when people are out of hospital – this is quite simple and many people learn to do it for themselves. There is a risk they can become infected though, so it's important to know the signs to watch for.

Oral chemotherapy

Some people may need to take oral chemotherapy as part of their regimen. You will probably collect the tablets or capsules from the day treatment unit. The person giving you the medicines should tell you what to take and when. This information will also be on the boxes or bottles containing your treatment.

Chemotherapy tablets or capsules should not be handled by anyone other than the person taking them. If you are a carer helping someone to take their chemotherapy, you should wear gloves when handling any tablets or capsules.

Intrathecal chemotherapy

Some kinds of high-grade lymphoma may involve the central nervous system or **CNS** (the brain and spinal cord). The CNS is surrounded by a fluid that cushions it called cerebrospinal fluid. It is also protected by something called the 'blood–brain barrier'. This stops many drugs crossing from the bloodstream into the cerebrospinal fluid.

One way to treat lymphoma in the CNS is to give chemotherapy directly into the cerebrospinal fluid. This is known as intrathecal chemotherapy.

Sometimes doctors also suggest giving intrathecal chemotherapy to prevent lymphoma spreading to the CNS in future. This is known as CNS **prophylaxis**. It is needed in only a small number of people where the risk of spread is high.

For more information about either lymphomas in the CNS or CNS prophylaxis please ring our helpline (0808 808 5555) or see our website (www.lymphomas.org.uk).

Intrathecal chemotherapy is usually given during a lumbar puncture. It is given by a senior doctor who is specially qualified to give intrathecal chemotherapy.

You will find more details about having a lumbar puncture on page 24.

Side effects of chemotherapy

It is not possible to say exactly what side effects you will have from your treatment. Everybody will notice slightly different side effects, even if they are having the same treatment as someone else.

The side effects of chemotherapy will depend on what drugs you are having. Your hospital team will give you information about what to expect.

We can provide more information about many of these side effects. Please see our website (www.lymphomas.org.uk) or ring our helpline (0808 808 5555) if you would like to know more or want to talk to someone about your side effects.

It is important to let your hospital team know about your side effects and whether any of them change. There are usually things that can be done to help.

Over the next few pages we describe some of the more common side effects of chemotherapy. There are side effects that could affect you during or soon after your treatment, and also side effects that could affect you later on, perhaps months or even years after your treatment.

→ You will find tips for coping with some of the common side effects of treatments for lymphoma in the appendix on pages 130–136.

Risk of infection and low blood cell counts

The most important side effect to know about is damage to the **bone marrow**. The job of your bone marrow is to make your body's blood cells. These include your **white blood cells** that help to fight infection. The most important white blood cell is called a **neutrophil**.

You may hear a low white cell count referred to as **neutropenia**, meaning the number of neutrophils is low. This happens quite commonly with many chemotherapy regimens used for high-grade lymphoma. It means you will be more at risk of infection. The white cell count tends to be lowest about 7–10 days after each dose of chemotherapy, but it can stay low for some time.

If you are neutropenic (have neutropenia), your chances of getting an infection are higher. If you develop an infection, it can be serious and sometimes it can even be life-threatening.

Call your hospital **at once** if you develop signs of an infection. These can include:
- fever
- temperature of 38°C or above (though your temperature might not be raised if you are taking steroid tablets; see pages 58–59)
- chills, shivering or sweating
- mouth sores and ulcers
- cough or sore throat
- redness or swelling of the skin, especially around your line if you have one or where you've had a cannula
- diarrhoea or abdominal pain
- burning sensation when passing urine
- feeling generally unwell or disorientated.

An infection in someone who has very low neutrophils needs to be treated urgently. This will usually mean going into hospital as an emergency for **intravenous** antibiotics. You should make sure you keep the contact numbers for your hospital handy at all times.

If you have to ring the hospital because you are not feeling well, do tell the person you speak to that you are having chemotherapy. If you are on a clinical trial, make sure you tell them about this too. That way they can make sure you get the best advice and get treatment quickly if you need it.

→ You will find some tips on how to lower your risk of infection if you are neutropenic on page 130.

Many people continue to feel well even though their **blood count** is low. If your white cell count is too low when your next cycle of treatment is due, your doctors may delay this until your blood count has had a chance to recover. You may need to have other drugs to help boost your blood cell count. These are called **growth factors** or **G-CSF**.

→ You will find more information about growth factors on pages 57–58.

Sometimes other blood cells can be affected by chemotherapy. Your **red blood cells** carry oxygen. A lack of these is called **anaemia**, which can make you feel tired or short of breath. Some people may need blood transfusions to ease their symptoms of anaemia.

Platelets help to stop you bleeding. A lack of platelets is called **thrombocytopenia**, which can make you more likely to bruise easily or bleed. People who are bleeding or have very low platelet counts are sometimes given a transfusion of platelets.

You will have regular blood tests taken to check your blood cell counts during your treatment.

Feeling sick
Some chemotherapy drugs can make you feel sick (or nauseous) after treatment. You might vomit too. You will be given anti-sickness drugs to help. These are called 'antiemetics'.

Tell your doctor or nurse if you are feeling sick. If you are taking anti-sickness drugs that aren't working, tell one of your hospital team. There are lots of different anti-sickness drugs and sometimes a change of drug is needed.

Sore mouth
Chemotherapy drugs may give you a sore mouth. This is because the chemotherapy damages the cells of the lining of your mouth. This is called 'mucositis' and can be painful. It can also make you more prone to mouth ulcers and infections. Your hospital team will be able to advise you about mouthwashes and painkillers that can help.

Change in taste and other dietary problems
It is quite common for people being treated with chemotherapy to have other problems with eating, such as:
- food tasting different or unpleasant
- loss of appetite.

> 'Chemo is no walk in the park, I had up days and down days, but it saved my life.'

Fatigue
Fatigue is one of the most common symptoms for people with lymphoma.

Cancer-related fatigue is quite different from normal tiredness. It can mean that you find it hard to concentrate or make decisions. It may make you short-tempered. You might sometimes feel too tired to do even simple things, like watching television. Fatigue can be difficult to describe and you may find that other people don't really understand it.

For more information about fatigue please ring our helpline (0808 808 5555) or see our website (www.lymphomas.org.uk).

It may be some months after treatment before your fatigue goes away. There is good evidence though that taking some regular gentle exercise can help people feel better more quickly.

> 'I was quite tired after each treatment. I tried to follow by body's signals and snoozed when I needed to.'

Hair loss
Some chemotherapy drugs used to treat high-grade lymphoma commonly cause hair loss. This means it is likely you will lose some or all of your hair. Hair loss will typically begin within a couple of weeks of starting treatment. It can fall out quite suddenly, which can be very distressing. Ask your team about wig facilities that are available on the NHS in your area or for advice on other headwear.

Your hair will usually start to grow back within a month or two of your treatment finishing. Sometimes it may seem different, perhaps curlier or a slightly different colour. It will probably take 6–12 months for it to return to its normal thickness.

→ You will find some tips for dealing with hair loss on pages 134–135.

Peripheral neuropathy
Some chemotherapy drugs cause damage to the nerves that carry information about touch, temperature and pain. The drugs can also damage other nerves, including the nerves involved in muscle movement. This nerve damage is called 'peripheral neuropathy'.

Peripheral neuropathy is usually due to certain groups of drugs. One drug often used in high-grade lymphoma that can cause neuropathy is vincristine (Oncovin®, the 'O' in CHOP).

Neuropathy commonly affects the nerves in your hands and feet, but you might feel it in other places too. Sometimes it can affect the nerves to the internal organs, which is known as 'autonomic neuropathy'.

It can cause:
- pins and needles
- pain
- numbness
- clumsiness
- problems with balance
- increased sensitivity to heat
- constipation
- temporary impotence.

Symptoms of neuropathy usually develop soon after you start treatment, but not everyone will get them.

If you have any of these symptoms, you should tell your doctors or nurses **before** you have your next dose of chemotherapy. They might want to make a change to your treatment to prevent these problems getting worse.

For most people, symptoms of peripheral neuropathy will be temporary, but some people can have long-term or permanent damage.

Bladder problems

The drugs cyclophosphamide (particularly in a high dose) and ifosfamide (Mitoxana®) can cause irritation and bleeding from the lining of the bladder and the kidneys. You will need to drink lots of fluid with these treatments and may also have extra fluid through your drip.

A drug called mesna can also be given to people having high doses of either ifosfamide or cyclophosphamide. Mesna can help to reduce problems with the bladder after chemotherapy. **Note:** if you notice blood in your urine, you should tell one of your hospital team straightaway.

Effects on fertility

Some treatments for lymphoma may reduce your fertility. Many people are able to have children after treatment without any problem, but certain chemotherapy drugs – especially the high-dose chemotherapy used in stem cell transplants – can make this less likely. Women closer to the age of normal menopause are more likely to have problems with fertility.

Your doctor will not be able to say for certain how your fertility might be affected, but they should talk about this with you before you start treatment.

Men may wish to think about sperm storage before they start treatment. Though being ill with lymphoma can reduce your sperm count even before you start treatment, developments in fertility treatment make sperm storage worthwhile for many men who may want to have children in the future.

The choices for women are more limited, partly because fertility treatments in women take more time. This could mean any lymphoma treatment is delayed, which may not be good for your health in the long term.

If this is an issue for you, you should talk to your team about seeing a specialist to find out more about what choices you have. Embryo storage may be possible for some women but it does take time. Egg storage and ovarian tissue freezing are not offered at all hospitals. At present, they are not as successful as sperm storage. Different hospitals will also have different policies about the funding of these treatments on the NHS.

Women may find that their periods become irregular or stop altogether during treatment. Afterwards their periods may return to normal but for some women, the irregularity continues when their treatment has finished. Some women, even those who remain fertile straight after treatment, may go through an **early menopause**.

Heart problems

Some drugs, especially doxorubicin (one of the drugs in CHOP), can cause damage to the heart, with problems sometimes developing many years later. You may have special tests such as an echocardiogram (often just called an 'echo') to see how well your heart is working before you start treatment.

Certain drugs may be avoided if your heart function is not good or if you have had heart trouble in the past. Even if your heart is normal, your doctors will be careful not to prescribe more than the safe maximum dose.

Blood problems
Some chemotherapy treatments can lead to a small increase in the risk of developing other blood problems in the future. These problems are very rare but can include myelodysplastic syndrome (MDS) or acute leukaemia.

MDS is an illness where the **bone marrow** no longer makes enough healthy blood cells. It can result in a low **blood count**, most often causing **anaemia** that may need to be treated with blood transfusions.

> Please ring our helpline if you would like to talk about the long-term side effects (late effects) of treatment (0808 808 5555).

Other treatments sometimes given with chemotherapy

Growth factors
Growth factors are copies of hormones that occur naturally in our body. They can help to keep the levels of your **white blood cells** up when you are having chemotherapy.

The growth factor most commonly used is called **G-CSF**. It triggers the bone marrow to make more stem cells, which can then become white blood cells. G-CSF is given as an injection into the fatty tissue under your skin (a **subcutaneous** injection). Most people learn to give the injections themselves or a relative may be taught how to give them. It is sometimes also possible for a nurse to give G-CSF at a GP surgery or even at home.

G-CSF can cause side effects such as flu-like symptoms, bone pain and headaches. If you feel unwell during your growth factor treatment, you should get in touch with your hospital straightaway.

Steroids

Steroids are drugs that mimic hormones made naturally by our bodies. The steroids used in lymphoma treatment help to kill the lymphoma cells. They also reduce nausea and help you to feel better. Steroids are usually given as tablets, often in the form of prednisolone.

Steroids can have many different side effects, including:
- weight gain – this is partly due to an increase in appetite and may be a good thing if you have been losing weight
- problems sleeping – you should usually try to take your steroids early in the day, if possible before lunchtime
- mood changes – you may feel more restless and irritable; some people find they have most problems on the days just after they have finished taking their steroids
- raised blood sugar – extra care may be needed to monitor your sugar levels if you have diabetes or a tendency towards it
- fluid retention, causing ankle swelling or puffiness of the hands and face
- infections – for example, you may be more likely to develop thrush (caused by candida infection) or cold sores (caused by a **virus**).

The side effects will depend on the dose used and whether the steroids are given for a short or long time.

Always tell your hospital team about any symptoms you have that might be side effects. There are often things that can be done to help. The side effects will improve once you stop taking the steroids.

> For more information about steroids please ring our helpline (0808 808 5555) or see our website (www.lymphomas.org.uk).

CHOP chemotherapy

The most commonly used chemotherapy **regimen** for high-grade non-Hodgkin lymphoma is known as CHOP. This is made up of three **intravenous** drugs – **c**yclophosphamide, **h**ydroxydaunorubicin (often known as doxorubicin) and vincristine (**O**ncovin®) – and oral **p**rednisolone tablets.

You usually don't need to stay in hospital to have this treatment – it is normally given in a day treatment unit. The intravenous drugs are given on the first day of each **cycle** and you will be given the prednisolone tablets to take at home for the first 5 days of each cycle.

This is followed by a rest period. You may still have other drugs to help prevent side effects during this time. Cycles of CHOP are usually given every 3 weeks.

Most people having CHOP for a B-cell lymphoma will also be given the antibody rituximab (MabThera®) on the first day of each cycle. The treatment is then known as R-CHOP.

→ You will find more information about rituximab on pages 61–62.

Other chemotherapy regimens
It is not possible to give details of all the regimens used to treat high-grade lymphoma in this booklet. You should be aware that if you are having a different treatment it may be quite unlike CHOP chemotherapy.

Your hospital team will give you full information about exactly how your treatment will be given. They will also be able to tell you what side effects you should expect from the drugs being used. Do ask your team if you are unsure about anything to do with your treatment.

→ If you would like to talk to someone about your chemotherapy please ring our helpline (0808 808 5555).

Antibody therapy

What is antibody therapy?
Antibodies are **proteins** in our blood that fight infection. They are made naturally by our bodies when we have an infection. They stick to proteins called 'antigens' on the surface of **bacteria** or **viruses** and tell our bodies to get rid of them.

Lymphoma cells have proteins on their surface too and these can be used as a target for treatment. Antibodies can be made in a laboratory to recognise these antigens. When the man-made antibody matches with and sticks to a lymphoma cell, it marks the cell out to be killed by the body's **immune system**.

Antibody therapy (sometimes called 'immunotherapy') is different from chemotherapy and radiotherapy because it targets cancer cells more directly. This means it does not have the same side effects as chemotherapy or radiotherapy.

The antibody most often used for high-grade lymphoma is called **rituximab** (or MabThera®). It targets an antigen called CD20. Because CD20 is found on **B lymphocytes** only, rituximab is mainly used to treat B-cell lymphomas.

Another antibody to CD20 known as **ofatumumab** (Arzerra®) is being used in trials too. Other new antibodies are also being developed and tested that target other proteins found on lymphoma cells.

How is antibody therapy given?
Rituximab for high-grade lymphoma is given together with chemotherapy. It is usually given at the start of each **cycle** of treatment. Rituximab is usually given to you as an outpatient, so you don't normally have to stay in hospital.

The first dose of rituximab is given as a drip (an infusion) into a vein. It must be given slowly to help prevent side effects. This may take a few hours.

After the first dose, further infusions may be given more quickly (over about an hour) if people have not had a bad reaction before.

In future it may be that further doses of rituximab for some people will be given as an injection into the layer of fat just under the skin (a **subcutaneous** injection). This means each dose can be given in about 5 minutes. Your doctor will let you know if this is suitable for you.

Side effects of antibody therapy

Most side effects of antibody therapy usually occur while the drip is being given (known as 'infusion-related side effects') rather than later on. They are more common with the first infusion and include shivers, fevers and other flu-like symptoms. When given subcutaneously, the skin where the injection was given may become red, swollen and painful. You will be given other drugs such as paracetamol and antihistamine to help reduce the chances of these problems.

Rarely, people have more serious side effects caused by an allergic reaction. If this happens, you may need to stay in hospital for a while as you recover. You may be able to have the infusion more slowly in future, or your doctor may decide it is best to avoid this treatment.

A very small number of people receiving rituximab have developed a viral brain infection known as PML (short for 'progressive multifocal leukoencephalopathy'). This is a serious complication but fortunately it is very rare.

> For more information about rituximab please ring our helpline (0808 808 5555) or see our website (www.lymphomas.org.uk).

Other targeted therapies

What are targeted therapies?

Targeted therapies are sometimes also called biological therapies. This is because they use specific 'biological' pathways to target the lymphoma cells.

More about treatments for high-grade non-Hodgkin lymphoma

The main kind of targeted therapy used in lymphoma is antibody therapy (see pages 60–62). Other kinds of targeted therapies are, however, now starting to be used for some types of high-grade lymphoma.

Many clinical trials are being done to test how well these new drugs work in different lymphomas. Some of these trials are being done in certain groups of people only, for example in older or less fit people.

Early results for some of the drugs look very promising. As a result they will probably be used more widely in the future. At present, doctors still need to know how and when it is best to use them.

There are different kinds of targeted drugs, which work in different ways. The following are some of the targeted drugs that are being used or tested in high-grade non-Hodgkin lymphoma.

Cell signal blockers

We now understand a lot more about the pathways within lymphoma cells that keep them alive or make them divide. Often signals reaching the surface of the cell trigger a series of steps along one or more pathways. Scientists have found that blocking either the signal or a key step in the pathway can make lymphoma cells die.

A number of new drugs have been developed to target these signals and pathways. **Ibrutinib** (see pages 81 and 89) is one such new drug that targets an important pathway in **B cells**. It is starting to be used in some B-cell lymphomas but trials are continuing to work out how best to use it.

Proteasome inhibitors

There are many **proteins** that help to control what happens in cells and how they divide. Proteasome inhibitors, such as **bortezomib** (Velcade®, see pages 81 and 89), upset the balance of these proteins. This seems to be particularly harmful to certain lymphoma cells, causing the cells to die.

Immunomodulators

Doctors think that these drugs work by changing (or 'modulating') how the immune system works. **Lenalidomide** (Revlimid®, see page 89) may do this in a number of ways. These include blocking some of the signals between immune system cells, blocking some of the signals inside lymphoma cells, and stopping new blood vessels growing in or around the lymphoma. The lymphoma cells are 'starved' of the support they need, so the lymphoma stops growing.

Antibody–drug conjugates

These are made up of an **antibody**, which targets the lymphoma cell, joined to a strong chemotherapy drug. This chemotherapy drug cannot simply be given into the bloodstream on its own because of its side effects. The antibody is able to deliver the drug directly to the lymphoma cells, thereby killing the lymphoma cells with fewer side effects.

These drugs include **brentuximab vedotin** (Adcetris®, see page 100), which is one new targeted drug already being used in certain types of lymphoma.

How are targeted therapies given?
This varies for different drugs but many of them are given by mouth (orally).

Brentuximab, like most antibodies, has to be given in a drip (an infusion) into a vein. Bortezomib was previously also given into a vein but is now available for injection just under the skin (a **subcutaneous** injection).

Lenalidomide and ibrutinib, like many of the newer targeted therapies, are taken as tablets. Usually these tablets are taken on many or all of the days in each **cycle**.

Side effects of targeted therapies
The side effects vary for different drugs. In general, targeted therapies often cause fewer side effects than standard chemotherapy.

They can make people feel more tired, especially if they are taking lenalidomide. Other side effects can include nausea or bowel upset. Hair loss is not generally a problem.

Most targeted therapies can affect the **bone marrow**, so there is still a risk of infection and bleeding. This is usually less of a problem than with most chemotherapy **regimens**. Both bortezomib and brentuximab can also cause peripheral neuropathy (see pages 53–54).

If your treatment includes a targeted therapy, your doctor will give you more information about what side effects to expect.

Radiotherapy

What is radiotherapy?
Radiotherapy uses high-energy X-rays, similar to those used to take an X-ray picture but given in much higher doses. The X-rays are directed to precise areas. They can kill off cancer cells in this area by stopping them dividing.

Radiotherapy is used for some people with high-grade non-Hodgkin lymphoma. Lymphoma cells are very sensitive to radiotherapy but the treatment can only be given to small areas.

It is therefore used to treat:
- localised (early-stage) lymphoma – most often after chemotherapy has been given
- people who have areas with very large **lymph nodes** (bulky disease) – this will be given after the full course of chemotherapy has been finished.

How is radiotherapy given?
A course of radiotherapy is given as a series of sessions known as 'fractions'. These are usually given daily, Monday to Friday, and you can go home after each treatment. The number of fractions will vary but treatment is often spread over a period of weeks.

Your radiotherapy care will be led by a clinical oncologist (or **radiotherapist**), who will talk with you about your treatment beforehand.

Treatment planning
This may involve more than one visit to the department before treatment starts. You will need to have a special

scan to produce a precise map of the area to be treated. This is then used to plan exactly where your radiotherapy will target.

The **radiographers** will need to make sure you are in exactly the same place on the treatment couch every time you have treatment, so they will mark dots on your skin to help. They will use a type of marker pen or will ask you if they can make some more permanent tiny ink marks on your skin. These are known as a 'radiotherapy tattoo' and will look like small freckles.

If you are having radiotherapy to the head or neck area, a shell will be made, usually from a plastic mesh. This will keep your head still and in the correct position. It also means you will not need any marks on your skin.

Having the treatment
During your treatment, the radiographers will position you carefully on the couch and ask you to stay very still. You will be in the treatment room for 10–20 minutes, but much of this time is spent getting you in exactly the right place. The actual treatment takes only a few minutes and you will not feel anything.

This kind of radiotherapy does not make you radioactive. There will be no risk to those close to you.

Side effects of radiotherapy
The side effects of radiotherapy will depend on what part of your body is being treated and the amount of radiotherapy given. You will be given information about what to expect and how to take care of yourself. You may find that you have no side effects to start with but

that they gradually become more obvious as you go through your course of treatment. They are often at their worst shortly after the treatment has finished, then start to improve.

Most radiotherapy side effects are short term and settle down. Some may be long term or permanent. Your doctors should talk about this with you before you start treatment.

> If you would like to talk about treatment side effects please ring our helpline (0808 808 5555).

It is important to let your hospital team know about your side effects. There are usually things that can be done to help. You may also be seen in a review clinic during your course of treatment.

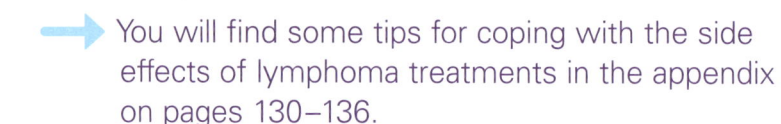

→ You will find some tips for coping with the side effects of lymphoma treatments in the appendix on pages 130–136.

Over the next few pages we will describe some of the more common side effects of radiotherapy.

Fatigue

Fatigue (extreme tiredness) is one of the most common symptoms for people with lymphoma. Fatigue is also a common side effect of radiotherapy. It may be many weeks or sometimes even a few months after treatment before you recover fully.

← You will find more information about fatigue on pages 52–53.

Sore skin

The skin in the area being treated may become pink, dry and itchy. If you have dark skin it might become darker. Rarely the skin can blister, a bit like sunburn. This is more likely to happen in folds of skin such as under the breast or in the groin. Skin reactions are usually at their worst a few days after the end of treatment and then start to heal.

You will be told how best to care for your skin. You may be asked to be careful when washing and drying the area. You may be given creams to keep the skin moisturised.

Hair loss

If you are having radiotherapy, hair loss or thinning should only occur in the area being treated. This hair loss will usually only be temporary. Your hair should start to grow back a few months after treatment.

Risk of infections and low blood counts

Radiotherapy may affect your **blood count**, particularly if certain bones are in the area being treated. If the white blood cell count falls (sometimes known as **neutropenia**), this can make you more prone to infections.

→ You will find some tips on how to lower your risk of infection if you are neutropenic on page 130.

You may also develop **anaemia**. This can make you feel tired and can also make you feel short of breath.

Sore mouth and problems swallowing
If you are having radiotherapy to the head, neck or upper chest, you may find that your mouth or throat becomes sore. You may also find that food starts to taste different or metallic.

If the area of the radiotherapy includes your salivary glands, your mouth will also become very dry. Your doctors may recommend artificial saliva or drugs to increase the amount of saliva you produce to help with this. It may take several months for this side effect to improve and sometimes it may be permanent.

If you are having radiotherapy to the chest or neck, you may also find that swallowing becomes a problem for a while.

Feeling sick
Sometimes radiotherapy can make you feel sick, in particular if your abdominal area is being treated. If you are feeling sick, tell the **radiographers**. It may help to have anti-sickness drugs (antiemetics) before each treatment starts. If you are taking anti-sickness drugs that aren't working, tell the radiographers. Sometimes a change in the anti-sickness drug is needed.

Lung problems
Lung fibrosis (scarring) can be a side effect of radiotherapy to the chest. Lung fibrosis, once it develops, is usually permanent. If mild it can be seen on X-rays or scans but will not cause you any symptoms. Some people can become short of breath and find they are able to do less exercise than before. The risk of this is lower if you do not smoke.

Heart disease and stroke

Radiotherapy to an area including the heart will increase your risk of heart disease in the future. This becomes more likely if you have had chemotherapy that also affects the heart. Treatment given to your chest and neck may also increase your risk of stroke in later life. These problems become more common 10 years or more after your treatment.

The risk of this happening to you will depend on the dose of radiotherapy and the exact area treated. You can help to lower the risk by taking good care of yourself, keeping your body at a healthy weight and giving up smoking. You should also see your doctor for advice about checking for high blood pressure, diabetes and high cholesterol.

Thyroid problems

Radiotherapy given to the neck can affect the thyroid gland, reducing the amount of the hormone thyroxine that it makes. A lack of thyroxine in the blood is called hypothyroidism. This may slow your metabolism, so you may feel very tired, gain weight easily or feel the cold more than normal.

Hypothyroidism can develop any time after treatment, even many years later. If you are at risk, a blood test to check your thyroid function should be done each year. If this shows your thyroid is becoming underactive, your GP will start you on thyroxine tablets.

There is also an increased risk of developing thyroid cancer many years after radiotherapy to the neck. This is very rare, however, unless you are treated at a young age.

Second cancers

Much of what is known about the higher risks of developing another cancer comes from clinical trials done many years ago in people with Hodgkin lymphoma. In these trials people were often treated with high doses of radiotherapy given to large areas of the body. Today people with high-grade lymphoma are given smaller doses of X-rays in a much more targeted way.

Your risk of developing a second cancer later on depends on the part of your body that is being treated:
- radiotherapy affecting the breast tissue in women, especially at a young age, increases the risk of breast cancer – regular breast screening is recommended from 8 years after the end of your radiotherapy onwards to detect any cancers early
- radiotherapy to the chest increases the risk of lung cancer – stopping smoking is vital to limit this risk.

Your doctor will be able to tell you what your risks are and offer you advice on what to do to reduce these risks.

> If you would like to talk to someone about the long-term effects (late effects) of treatment, please ring our helpline (0808 808 5555).

Stem cell transplants

Some people with high-grade non-Hodgkin lymphoma may be offered treatment with a stem cell transplant:
- people with **relapsed** lymphoma
- people who are thought to be at high risk of relapse
- people whose lymphoma has not responded to the standard treatment.

A stem cell transplant may work when standard treatments have not cured, or are thought to be unlikely to cure, someone's lymphoma. Stem cells are special cells normally found in the **bone marrow** that produce new blood cells. The stem cells used in a transplant may be either **autologous** (your own cells) or **allogeneic** (a donor's cells).

Stem cell transplants for high-grade lymphoma are usually autologous. This is a way of giving a much higher dose of treatment to your lymphoma. Allogeneic transplants are more complex and are less often done for high-grade lymphoma.

Stem cell transplants carry risks as well as benefits. This means they are not suitable for everyone. Most people having a transplant need to stay in hospital for some weeks and recovery can take many months. If your doctors are thinking about this form of treatment for you, they will talk to you in detail about it.

> We produce a booklet about autologous stem cell transplants for lymphoma. Please ring our helpline (0808 808 5555) or see our website (www.lymphomas.org.uk) if you would like a copy. We also have more information about allogeneic transplants if your doctors suggest this as a possible treatment for you.

Key facts

Chemotherapy
Chemotherapy means drug treatment. Often a combination of drugs is given together, known as a regimen. The drugs are given in treatment 'cycles'. Each cycle usually includes a rest period too, which allows the healthy cells in the body time to recover.

Treatment usually takes several months to finish.

Chemotherapy is usually given into a vein (intravenously) and/or as tablets (orally). For most people with high-grade lymphoma it will be given to you as an outpatient.

There are lots of possible side effects of treatment. Your side effects will depend on what kind of treatment you are having. You will be given information about what side effects to expect.

If you develop signs of infection or notice side effects, you should tell the team at the hospital at once. There are usually things that can be done to help. An infection in someone who has low neutrophils needs to be treated urgently.

Antibody therapy
Antibody therapy is given with chemotherapy for some high-grade lymphomas. It works by sticking to a protein on the lymphoma cell. The antibody marks the lymphoma cell out to be killed by the body's immune system.

The antibody therapy most commonly used for non-Hodgkin lymphoma is rituximab (MabThera®). Antibody therapy is usually given as an intravenous infusion. It will normally be given to you as an outpatient.

Flu-like symptoms during the infusion are the commonest side effect. You will be given drugs to prevent these.

Other targeted therapies

Targeted therapies work in a number of different ways. They may use antibodies to carry another treatment directly to the lymphoma cells. They may block the signals in or around the lymphoma cells that help them grow.

Targeted therapies often have fewer side effects than other treatments. Many of them are taken as tablets.

Lots of clinical trials are being done to look at how best to use targeted therapies. Early results for some of these drugs look very promising.

Radiotherapy

Radiotherapy for high-grade lymphoma is most often given after chemotherapy.

Your radiotherapy care will be led by a clinical oncologist (or radiotherapist). You will visit the department so that your treatment can be carefully planned beforehand.

Radiotherapy is painless. Each fraction (session) of treatment takes 10–20 minutes in total. It usually continues for several weeks.

The side effects of radiotherapy will depend on the area being treated as well as the total amount given. They tend to develop towards the end of treatment. You should be given information about what side effects to expect.

If you notice side effects, tell your hospital team about these as there are often things that can be done to help.

Types of high-grade non-Hodgkin lymphoma

B-cell non-Hodgkin lymphomas

T-cell non-Hodgkin lymphomas

Non-Hodgkin lymphomas associated with immunodeficiency

High-grade non-Hodgkin lymphoma

This part of the booklet looks in more detail at the most common types of high-grade lymphoma.

⬅ You will find a list of the lymphomas in this section in the contents on pages 7–8.

We would suggest that, at least at first, you read only the section on your own type of high-grade lymphoma.

If you are not sure exactly what kind of lymphoma you have, check this with your doctor. It may be confusing or distressing to read about illnesses that are not relevant to you.

We have not been able to give details of every type of high-grade non-Hodgkin lymphoma. If you have been told you have a type of lymphoma that you do not see listed in this booklet, you may wish to check with your doctor. They may have used another name for a lymphoma that is included. If not, they might be able to tell you if there is a lymphoma included that is close to yours.

For each lymphoma we are aiming to answer these questions:
- What does the name mean?
- Who typically gets it?
- How might it affect me?
- How might it be treated?

B-cell non-Hodgkin lymphomas

Diffuse large B-cell lymphoma

What does it mean?
Diffuse large B-cell lymphoma (DLBCL) is the most common kind of high-grade non-Hodgkin lymphoma. Almost 1 in every 3 people with non-Hodgkin lymphoma will have DLBCL.

The name describes the type of cell involved and its appearance. So it is a lymphoma formed from **B cells** that are large compared with the cells seen in other lymphomas. The cells have a 'diffuse' pattern, meaning they are spread throughout the **lymph node** and have replaced its normal structure.

Experts now know that not all DLBCLs are the same. Some types have developed from a slightly more mature B cell. Research studies have shown two main types, known as the GCB (germinal centre B cell) and ABC (activated B cell) types. Scientists are now beginning to understand a lot more about what makes the cells in each of these lymphoma types grow. Knowing this is helping doctors to design clinical trials using some of the newer targeted drugs. These may result in treatments that work even better in future and may allow these targeted treatments to be given to those who will get most benefit.

> We have some further information about DLBCL on our website (www.lymphomas.org.uk). You can also ask for a copy of this information from our helpline (0808 808 5555).

Who gets it?

DLBCL is slightly more common in men than in women. It can develop in people of any age, but is more likely to occur in people aged over 50.

Sometimes, DLBCL develops in people who are known to have low-grade (slow-growing) non-Hodgkin lymphoma. The low-grade lymphoma can change (or 'transform') into DLBCL.

How will it affect me?

Some people have no symptoms; most have a lump or swelling that is easily felt. You may have more general symptoms such as weight loss, flu-like symptoms, night sweats or tiredness.

Other symptoms of DLBCL will depend on what part of your body is involved. It is quite common for people with DLBCL to have **extranodal** lymphoma. For example, DLBCL may involve the bowel, causing symptoms such as abdominal pain and diarrhoea.

Some people with DLBCL have localised lymphoma (stage I or II) at the time of **diagnosis**. Most people will have more advanced lymphoma (stage III or IV). This may sound alarming but there are good treatments available for DLBCL whatever its stage.

⬅ You will find more about the stages of lymphoma on pages 25–26.

How will it be treated?

The treatment of your DLBCL depends on the stage of your lymphoma, as well as your age and general health.

Most patients will have a combination of chemotherapy and antibody therapy. The most commonly used **regimen** is R-CHOP (see page 59).

Radiotherapy is a good treatment for lymphoma but it can only be given to a small area.

Early-stage DLBCL can be treated with a limited number of **cycles** of chemotherapy (for example, four cycles of R-CHOP) and then radiotherapy to the area where the lymphoma was.

More advanced DLBCL will usually be treated with more cycles of chemotherapy (typically six to eight cycles of R-CHOP). Radiotherapy is then usually only given if, before the chemotherapy, there were areas where the lymph nodes were very large – this is sometimes referred to as having 'bulky' disease.

Clinical trials are looking at whether treatment for DLBCL can be made better for certain people by adding one of the newer targeted therapies to R-CHOP. Doctors think that adding in targeted therapies, such as bortezomib (Velcade®) or ibrutinib, might make R-CHOP work better in people with the ABC type. Clinical trials are underway, and depending on the results, the treatments for the GCB and ABC types may differ slightly in future.

Some people with DLBCL will also need treatment to the **CNS** (the brain and spinal cord). Spread to the CNS is more common when DLBCL occurs at certain **extranodal** sites, such as the testes, breasts or sinuses.

If lymphoma is found in your CNS, you may need to have other chemotherapy regimens instead of R-CHOP, and/or intrathecal chemotherapy.

← You will find more details about intrathecal chemotherapy on pages 47–48.

If there is no lymphoma in your CNS at present but your doctors think it could spread there later, you may be offered extra treatment. This preventive treatment aims to reduce the risk of your lymphoma spreading to your CNS. It is known as CNS **prophylaxis**.

For more information about preventive therapy for the central nervous system in lymphoma (CNS prophylaxis) please ring the helpline (0808 808 5555) or see our website (www.lymphomas.org.uk).

Some people who have DLBCL that is not thought to have been cured after R-CHOP may be offered further treatment. This will usually include a stem cell transplant if people are fit enough.

Burkitt lymphoma

What does it mean?
Burkitt lymphoma is named after a doctor called Denis Burkitt, who first wrote about this kind of cancer in children and young adults in Africa. The name is now also used for a similar fast-growing type of lymphoma that is seen in other parts of the world too.

Who gets it?
Burkitt lymphoma can affect both children and adults, but it is quite rare, especially in older adults. More than a third of children who develop lymphoma have this kind.

People who are infected with **HIV** are more likely to develop Burkitt lymphoma.

Although Burkitt lymphoma mainly affects people who do not have HIV, your doctors will recommend you have a test to rule out this infection. This is because HIV is now treatable and, if found, you would need treatment for both HIV and lymphoma at the same time.

How will it affect me?
Because Burkitt lymphoma is fast growing, your symptoms may have developed over just a few days or weeks.

It usually causes lots of large **lymph nodes** in many different parts of the body, including the chest, the tonsils and the back of the nose and throat. Burkitt lymphoma can also be found in other organs, such as the **spleen** and the liver. Many people will have lymphoma in their **bone marrow** at the time they are diagnosed.

You may also have the other symptoms of lymphoma, including night sweats, tiredness, flu-like symptoms and weight loss.

Compared with other lymphomas, Burkitt lymphoma is more likely to affect your bowel and the lymph nodes in your abdomen. People with Burkitt lymphoma often go to their doctor with abdominal pain, nausea, vomiting and diarrhoea. It can also cause a collection of fluid within your abdomen (called 'ascites') or may cause your bowel to become obstructed or bleed.

Burkitt lymphoma is more likely to involve your brain and spinal cord (the **CNS**) than other lymphomas.

Burkitt lymphoma in children often affects the jaw. The lymphoma commonly grows in the areas where permanent teeth are forming.

How is it treated?

Many people with Burkitt lymphoma can be cured using a combination of strong chemotherapy drugs. A commonly used **regimen** is CODOX-M, which may be used with IVAC. These initials refer to the names of the individual drugs.

This type of chemotherapy can only be given to inpatients. It is usually given through a tunnelled central line.

⬅ You will find some information about central lines on pages 46–47.

CODOX-M on its own is used for people with early-stage Burkitt lymphoma who haven't yet become too unwell.

CODOX-M/IVAC is used for people with more advanced-stage Burkitt lymphoma. Often a large number of lymphoma cells are killed very quickly when this type of therapy is started. This can cause problems, particularly with your kidneys, so the drug rasburicase (Fasturtec®) is sometimes used to protect the kidneys.

Rituximab is now added to chemotherapy for Burkitt lymphoma as this has been shown to make the treatment more effective.

⬅ You will find more information about rituximab on pages 61–62.

These regimens are strong chemotherapy and your doctors may be worried you are not fit enough for them. If this is the case, they may suggest a slightly more gentle chemotherapy regimen instead.

Because Burkitt lymphoma commonly involves the CNS, all patients with Burkitt lymphoma need to have treatment that can reach their CNS. The regimens mentioned here use drugs that can enter the CNS from the bloodstream and also drugs that are given intrathecally (directly into the cerebrospinal fluid).

⬅ You will find more about intrathecal chemotherapy on pages 47–48.

📞 For more information on CNS lymphoma and its treatment please ring our helpline (0808 808 5555) or see our website (www.lymphomas.org.uk).

The chemotherapy typically used for Burkitt lymphoma is stronger than many other regimens, so most people spend quite long spells in hospital. This is so that the right care can be given during and after treatment and any side effects can be properly treated. Most people spend a bit of time at home between each **cycle** but the full treatment takes several months to finish.

Mantle cell lymphoma

What does it mean?
Mantle cell lymphoma (MCL) is an uncommon type of non-Hodgkin lymphoma. The word 'mantle' is used because the lymphoma cells come from a part of the **lymph node** called the 'mantle zone'.

Although mantle cell lymphoma usually looks like a low-grade (slow-growing) lymphoma under the microscope, it often doesn't behave this way. Some mantle cell lymphomas do grow slowly, but others grow more rapidly and need early and often intensive treatment.

Who gets it?
MCL makes up about 1 in 20 of all non-Hodgkin lymphomas.

It is more common in men than it is in women. It is more likely to affect older people, typically people in their 60s.

How will it affect me?
Most people with MCL go to their doctor because they notice big lymph nodes. By the time this happens and the **diagnosis** is made, most people already have advanced-stage lymphoma (stage III or IV).

MCL very commonly involves the bowel. This could give you symptoms such as diarrhoea and abdominal pain.

MCL usually involves the **bone marrow**. The presence of lots of lymphoma cells in the bone marrow can stop it making healthy blood cells.

Types of high-grade non-Hodgkin lymphoma

This can cause **anaemia**, which can make you feel short of breath and very tired. The number of **platelets** in your blood might also be reduced. This would make you more likely to bleed or to bruise very easily.

The lymphoma cells are sometimes found in the bloodstream too. This can be a good sign if your **spleen** is also bigger than normal and you don't have big lymph nodes. It means your lymphoma is more likely to be a slower-growing type of MCL.

How is it treated?
Until recently MCL has been hard to treat successfully, but many new treatments are now being developed. It is, however, not likely you will be cured of MCL. Your doctors will instead be aiming to get your lymphoma into as good a remission as possible, for as long as possible. The exact treatment that is chosen for you will depend on your own circumstances, for instance how fit you are.

If you feel relatively well, you may have no active treatment until your symptoms become harder to live with. Doctors suggest this more often to people who have lymphoma cells in their blood and a big spleen. Delaying active treatment like this means you will avoid having side effects. It also saves the treatments until you really need them. This is known as the 'watch-and-wait' approach and is used in a number of low-grade lymphomas.

> If you would like to find out more or talk to someone about watch and wait please ring our helpline (0808 808 5555) or see our website (www.lymphomas.org.uk).

When MCL needs to be treated, you will most likely have a chemotherapy **regimen** including several drugs. Your doctor will think about which of the treatments for MCL is best for you as there are a number of choices. Some are very strong chemotherapy treatments that may mean you have to stay in hospital to have them.

Rituximab is also given with chemotherapy as this makes the treatment work better. If you are not going to have a stem cell transplant after your chemotherapy, you may also be offered 'maintenance' rituximab therapy. This means rituximab continues to be given once every 2–3 months. This should mean your MCL stays in remission for longer.

If you are younger and fit, your doctors may also talk to you about having a stem cell transplant. Results from trials suggest this is the best way of giving you a long remission. But transplants carry many risks and side effects, so they are not suitable for everyone. Your doctors will talk to you in more detail if they think this could be the best treatment for you.

← You will find more information about stem cell transplants on pages 72–73.

Sometimes more gentle tablet chemotherapy will be used to treat MCL. The drugs used include:
- chlorambucil (Leukeran®)
- cyclophosphamide
- fludarabine (Fludara®).

The **intravenous** drug bendamustine (Levact®) is also quite often used to treat MCL.

There are a number of new targeted treatments for MCL that have been, and continue to be, tested in clinical trials. These include:
- lenalidomide (Revlimid®)
- bortezomib (Velcade®)
- ibrutinib.

Mostly the trials of these new drugs have been done in people who have already had a number of other treatments. Early results have looked promising and some of these drugs will hopefully be available in the next few years.

You might also like to ask your doctor whether there is a trial suitable for you.

Primary mediastinal large B-cell lymphoma

What does it mean?
Primary mediastinal large B-cell lymphoma (PMBL) is a type of diffuse large B-cell lymphoma (DLBCL) that particularly involves the **lymph nodes** in the mediastinum. The mediastinum is the area of the chest between the lungs. It contains the heart, the windpipe, the oesophagus (where food goes down) and other structures including lymph nodes, the thymus gland and major blood vessels. PMBL is believed to start in **B cells** within the thymus.

Who gets it?
PMBL makes up around 1 in 50 of all non-Hodgkin lymphomas. It affects younger people, typically between the ages of 20 and 40. It is twice as common in women.

How will it affect me?
PMBL involves the lymph nodes in the chest. These can sometimes grow very big, which is known as having bulky disease. You may have a cough, shortness of breath and problems breathing. Very big lymph nodes can sometimes make these symptoms quite severe.

You may also have other symptoms of lymphoma, such as fever, night sweats and weight loss.

How is it treated?
PMBL is treated with chemotherapy and antibody therapy. The treatment used most often is R-CHOP (see page 59).

If the nodes in your chest are very large, you may have radiotherapy to this area after your other treatment. The treatments given for PMBL usually work very well. Your chances of being cured are high.

Primary central nervous system lymphoma (including primary intraocular lymphoma)

What does it mean?
Non-Hodgkin lymphomas can affect almost any part of the body, including the brain and spinal cord, which is known as the central nervous system (**CNS**).

Lymphoma can involve the CNS in a number of ways. A lymphoma that starts within the CNS is known as a 'primary central nervous system lymphoma' (PCNSL). Lymphoma can also spread to the CNS from other parts of the body (secondary CNS lymphoma) or can affect the CNS by pressing on it from outside.

One particular part of the CNS that can be affected by lymphoma is the eye. Lymphoma in the eye is known as 'primary intraocular lymphoma' (PIOL). The lymphoma may affect only the eye or might affect other parts of the CNS too.

> For more information on CNS lymphoma please ring our helpline (0808 808 5555) or see our website (www.lymphomas.org.uk).

Who gets it?
PCNSL is a very rare lymphoma, making up less than 1 in every 100 non-Hodgkin lymphomas. It is slightly more common in men. It is more common in people aged 50–70.

It is more common in people whose **immune system** is not working. In the past it was common in people with **HIV** but better treatments for HIV have now made it less common.

How will it affect me?
PCNSL can affect a person in many different ways. Sometimes the lymphoma forms a lump that presses on part of the CNS. The exact symptoms this causes depend on the area involved. Sometimes the lymphoma will spread along the meninges (the layers of tissue that surround the CNS). You might hear this referred to as 'lymphomatous meningitis'.

Possible symptoms of PCNSL include headaches, changes in vision, drowsiness, problems with memory or balance, seizures (fits), muscle weakness, changes in personality or problems with speech.

People with PCNSL are likely to become more confused and have problems with understanding.

Surprisingly, people with PIOL do not always have problems with their eyesight at first.

How is it treated?
PCNSL is a difficult lymphoma to treat successfully. This is partly because people with PCNSL are often very sick by the time the lymphoma is found. This means treatment needs to be planned on an individual basis.

As this is a rare lymphoma, you may need to be cared for at a specialist cancer centre. The doctors there are likely to have seen more people with this type of lymphoma. They are also more likely to offer clinical trials that you may wish to take part in. Even if you choose not to be treated there, you may at least wish to be seen by the doctors to get their advice on your treatment choices.

Most people will have treatment with steroids – often the drug dexamethasone is chosen. The steroids can make the lymphoma shrink, at least for a while. They also help to reduce the swelling of the brain around the lymphoma. This can help to relieve symptoms in the short term. It may also help to make people fitter so that they can then have other treatments.

If you are fit enough, you will probably be offered chemotherapy. Chemotherapy for PCNSL involves high doses of the few drugs that are able to reach the CNS from the bloodstream (usually methotrexate together with cytarabine). These are given **intravenously** as an infusion (drip) and you will need to be an inpatient. Not all hospitals will be able to give these treatments so you may need to go to a larger centre.

Radiotherapy may be given to the eye for PIOL. It may also be given to the brain for PCNSL. In this case it probably needs to be given after chemotherapy if the aim is to cure the lymphoma. It is sometimes used on its own though when the aim is just to relieve symptoms and control the lymphoma for a while.

Large doses of radiotherapy may not be suitable for everyone, in particular people who already have symptoms such as confusion or problems with understanding. These symptoms and others such as memory loss can sometimes worsen or even occur for the first time after radiotherapy. This is most likely to happen if you are over the age of 60 or if you have had chemotherapy before. Your doctor should talk with you about all these risks before you start treatment.

← You will find information about other possible side effects of radiotherapy on pages 67–72.

Occasionally high-dose therapy and a stem cell transplant may be possible for people with PCNSL. But this will be suitable for only a small number of people, generally those who are younger, fitter and have done well with earlier therapy.

Clinical trials continue to test which treatments are best for people with PCNSL and PIOL.

T-cell non-Hodgkin lymphomas

Lymphoblastic lymphoma

What does it mean?
Lymphoblastic lymphoma (LBL) grows from a **lymphocyte** that is known as a 'lymphoblast'. This is a type of lymphocyte that is at an early stage of development. It is sometimes just called a 'blast'.

LBLs are in many ways like acute leukaemia. In lymphoma the blasts form lumps in the lymphatic system; in contrast, in leukaemia they grow mainly in the **bone marrow** and the blood. In practice, they often have the same effect on the body. There can also be blasts in the bone marrow and in the blood in LBL, just like an acute leukaemia.

LBL can grow from either **B cells** or **T cells**. T-cell LBL is more common than B-cell LBL.

Who gets it?
LBL affects young people, typically in their late teens or 20s. It is more common in men.

How will it affect me?
LBL grows very quickly. You may find that the symptoms develop within a few weeks.

LBL very often results in a large lump of lymphoma that grows from the **lymph nodes** in the mediastinum. The mediastinum is the area of the chest between the lungs. It contains the heart, the windpipe, the oesophagus (where food goes down) and other structures, including the major blood vessels and the thymus gland (where T cells mature).

If the lymph nodes in the mediastinum are big enough they may squash the structures in your mediastinum. This may make you cough, feel short of breath or have problems with your blood circulation.

Sometimes large nodes in the mediastinum are seen when a chest X-ray is done and lymphoma may not have been suspected beforehand.

LBL can also damage the pleura (the layers surrounding your lungs). This can cause pain in your chest when you breathe. It sometimes causes fluid to collect around your lung, known as a 'pleural effusion'.

You may also have other symptoms of lymphoma, including night sweats, tiredness, flu-like symptoms and weight loss.

As with leukaemia, you may have problems because your **bone marrow** is involved. This is because having lots of lymphoma cells in the bone marrow stops it making healthy blood cells.

This can result in **anaemia**, which can make you feel short of breath and very tired. The number of **platelets** in your blood might also be reduced. This means you are more likely to bleed or to bruise very easily.

LBL can also involve the **CNS** (the brain and spinal cord).

How is it treated?

LBL is treated with the same kind of chemotherapy as acute leukaemia. This treatment takes longer than most lymphoma treatments. It is split into different phases.

The first phase is called 'remission induction'. This is treatment that aims to get rid of all the lumps of lymphoma that can be seen on scans. It involves having a mixture of chemotherapy drugs given both in a drip into a vein (an infusion) and as tablets. This phase usually lasts several weeks, but it will depend on your exact **regimen**. You will have to stay in hospital for much of this time.

The next phase is called 'consolidation'. This aims to kill off any lymphoma cells that are still about, even though there are no longer any lumps to see. Consolidation involves having chemotherapy with a different combination of drugs. You usually don't have to stay in hospital during this time but the whole phase lasts a few months.

The third phase of treatment is called 'maintenance'. This involves mostly taking chemotherapy tablets but occasionally having more intravenous chemotherapy. Maintenance treatment lasts for 2 years.

Some people may be offered high-dose therapy followed by a stem cell transplant instead of having maintenance therapy.

For more information on stem cell transplants please ring our helpline (0808 808 5555) or see our website (www.lymphomas.org.uk).

Most people with LBL also have chemotherapy treatment to the brain and spinal cord (the **CNS**). This will help to treat any lymphoma that is in the CNS now, or to prevent it spreading there in the future. This treatment is known as CNS **prophylaxis** and usually includes intrathecal chemotherapy.

⬅ You will find more information about intrathecal chemotherapy on pages 47–48.

📞 For more information on CNS prophylaxis please ring our helpline (0808 808 5555) or see our website (www.lymphomas.org.uk).

Peripheral T-cell lymphoma

What does it mean?
Peripheral T-cell lymphoma (PTCL) covers a group of similar lymphomas. The word 'peripheral' means that the **T cells** have developed in parts of the body peripheral to (or outside of) the thymus gland.

Who gets it?
PTCL makes up around 1 in 13 of all non-Hodgkin lymphomas. It is a lymphoma that occurs in adults, more often in people over the age of 50. It affects more men than women.

How will it affect me?
Most people will have advanced-stage high-grade lymphoma (stage III or IV) by the time they go to their doctor. The **lymph nodes** often grow only a little bigger than normal but they occur in many areas of the body. You may also have night sweats, fevers and weight loss.

It is quite common for the liver and **spleen** to be involved and to become much larger than normal. PTCL often affects the **bone marrow** too. Your skin may also be affected, causing itchy red patches.

How is it treated?
PTCL is usually treated with chemotherapy, typically CHOP (see page 59). In younger patients, the treatment may be continued after this and may include a stem cell transplant.

PTCL can be hard to treat successfully with standard chemotherapy. If your lymphoma does not respond to CHOP or comes back after treatment, you may be offered other chemotherapy **regimens**. These often include gemcitabine (Gemzar®).

If you are otherwise fit, an **allogeneic** stem cell transplant may be another possible treatment. A number of new drugs are becoming available. You may also be asked if you would like to take part in a clinical trial.

Anaplastic large cell lymphoma

What does it mean?
Anaplastic large cell lymphoma (ALCL) is a lymphoma that develops from a **T cell**. The cells are large when looked at under a microscope and the word 'anaplastic' means 'disordered growth'.

Experts have now divided ALCL into two different types, depending on whether or not a certain protein is found on the cells. The type with the **protein** has a change affecting the genes of its cells.

This change in the genes creates a protein called ALK (anaplastic large-cell kinase). The cause of this change is unknown. Doctors refer to the type of ALCL with the change as 'ALK-positive ALCL'. The other type is called 'ALK-negative ALCL'.

Who gets it?
ALCL makes up around 3 out of every 100 non-Hodgkin lymphomas. The ALK-positive type tends to affect younger adults or children and is more common in men and boys.

ALK-negative ALCL is also more common in men but is seen in older adults, most commonly between the ages of 40 and 65.

How will it affect me?
As well as affecting **lymph nodes**, ALK-positive ALCL often affects **extranodal** sites, such as bones, skin, lungs and liver. You may also have other symptoms of lymphoma, including fevers, sweats and weight loss.

ALK-negative ALCL tends to be fast growing and can also sometimes involve extranodal sites such as the skin. When it involves the skin, it causes itchy red patches that are raised and scaly. Sometimes it is found only in the skin – this is called 'primary cutaneous ALCL'.

How is it treated?
ALCL is often treated with CHOP chemotherapy, but ALK-negative ALCL usually responds less well to this.

⬅ You will find more information about CHOP chemotherapy on page 59.

If you have ALK-negative ALCL and are fit enough, you may instead be offered a stronger chemotherapy **regimen** and possibly a stem cell transplant.

People with very large lymph nodes may be offered treatment with radiotherapy too.

The new targeted drug called brentuximab (Adcetris®) seems to be a useful treatment for ALCL. It worked well in a clinical trial for people with ALCL that was **refractory** or had **relapsed**.

← You will find further information about brentuximab (a type of antibody–drug conjugate) on pages 64–65.

Clinical trials will now be done to look at whether it should be used as part of the first course of treatment too. You may like to ask your doctor whether there is a suitable trial for you.

If you have primary cutaneous ALK-negative ALCL (where the lymphoma is in your skin only) it may get better without treatment.

When skin lymphoma needs treatment, the choices may be quite different. We produce information specifically about skin (cutaneous) lymphomas. Please see our website (www.lymphomas.org.uk) or ring our helpline (0808 808 5555) if you need this information.

Angioimmunoblastic T-cell lymphoma

What does it mean?
Angioimmunoblastic T-cell lymphoma (AITL) is a rare T-cell non-Hodgkin lymphoma. The term 'angio' refers to blood vessels – new blood vessels often grow in an abnormal pattern in lumps of AITL.

AITL seems to be linked to a past infection with the Epstein–Barr virus (EBV). The reason EBV infection causes this rare lymphoma in a few people is not yet clear.

Who gets it?
AITL makes up around 1 in every 100 non-Hodgkin lymphomas. It is more common in people aged over 60. It affects more men than women.

How will it affect me?
AITL can produce a wide range of symptoms and often people feel generally unwell.

It is likely you will have large **lymph nodes** in many areas of your body. Your liver and **spleen** may also be larger than normal. The other symptoms of lymphoma – fevers, itching, weight loss and night sweats – are common in people with AITL too.

Unlike in many other lymphomas, the cancerous cells of AITL produce abnormal **proteins**. These proteins can cause your body's **immune system** to react against your own cells. This is known as an 'autoimmune' reaction and it can cause a rash, painful joints, pins and needles and numbness.

How is it treated?
AITL is hard to treat successfully. The usual first treatment is CHOP chemotherapy (see page 59). If you are not well enough for this, you will probably have steroids. These can help to control your lymphoma and improve your symptoms. If they help, you may later be able to have chemotherapy too.

It is common for AITL to relapse after treatment with CHOP. To make this less likely, some people might continue to take a low dose of chemotherapy after finishing CHOP.

If the lymphoma does come back, other chemotherapy using different drugs, such as gemcitabine (Gemzar®), can be offered. Some people may be offered treatment with a stem cell transplant. New treatments also continue to be tested for AITL.

← You will find more about stem cell transplants on pages 72–73.

Enteropathy-associated T-cell lymphoma

What does it mean?
Enteropathy-associated T-cell lymphoma (EATL) grows in the small bowel (part of our intestines). 'Enteropathy' means a disease that causes wasting of the lining of the intestines, especially the small bowel.

Who gets it?
EATL is a rare lymphoma. Fewer than 1 in every 100 non-Hodgkin lymphomas will be of this type.

This lymphoma is linked to coeliac disease. Sometimes coeliac disease is diagnosed at the same time as the lymphoma.

Coeliac disease is caused by an abnormal reaction (sensitivity) to a protein called 'gluten' that is found in wheat and in some other grains. Eating foods that contain gluten results in damage to the lining of the small bowel. This damage causes diarrhoea, abdominal pain and weight loss.

EATL only develops in a tiny fraction of people who have coeliac disease. Rarely, EATL occurs on its own, without there being any sign of coeliac disease.

How will it affect me?
EATL causes bowel and stomach problems, so you may have diarrhoea, abdominal pain and weight loss. It can also cause ulcers in the bowel and may occasionally cause the bowel to perforate.

EATL can also cause **lymph nodes** to swell in other areas of the body. You may have night sweats and fevers too.

Because it looks like many other diseases of the bowel, EATL can be hard to diagnose. Other more common diseases are likely to be ruled out before lymphoma is thought of. It can also be tricky to get good pictures of the bowel using standard scans. For these reasons, people with EATL have often been unwell for some time before it is diagnosed.

How is it treated?
The usual treatment for EATL is CHOP chemotherapy. Coeliac disease is usually treated by eating a special gluten-free diet.

EATL can be hard to treat successfully. You may be offered other kinds of chemotherapy if CHOP does not give a good response. Sometimes people with EATL will be offered high-dose therapy and a stem cell transplant.

In some cases, people will have an operation to remove the affected parts of the bowel. Most people then go on to have chemotherapy to reduce the chances of **relapse** in other areas.

Adult T-cell leukaemia/lymphoma

What does it mean?
Adult T-cell leukaemia/lymphoma (ATLL) is a rare type of lymphoma that develops from a **T cell**.

In some people the lymphoma cells are found in the **bone marrow** and blood. This is why the term 'leukaemia' is included in the name of this lymphoma.

Who gets it?
ATLL is one of the types of lymphoma that is linked to a specific **virus**. The virus is known as HTLV-1 and is common in Japan, South-East Asia, the Caribbean, south-eastern USA, South America and parts of Africa.

As a result, ATLL is found most often in these parts of the world. It is much less common in the UK, where it is seen mainly in people of Afro-Caribbean origin.

Most people who develop ATLL are around the age of 50–60.

How will it affect me?
The symptoms of ATLL are varied. Some people have no symptoms or notice just a single lump.

Other people will have more symptoms such as lots of large **lymph nodes**, night sweats, fevers and a rash. These may come on very rapidly.

ATLL very commonly involves the bone marrow. Having lots of lymphoma cells in the bone marrow can stop it making healthy blood cells. This can result in **anaemia**, which can make you feel short of breath and very tired. The number of **platelets** in your blood might also be reduced. This means you are more likely to bleed or to bruise easily.

ATLL commonly causes high levels of calcium in the blood, known as 'hypercalcaemia'. This can cause many symptoms, such as nausea, constipation, weakness, tiredness and confusion. It can also sometimes cause serious problems with the heart and kidneys so must be treated quickly.

As well as causing large lymph nodes, ATLL can involve the liver and **spleen**, making these larger than normal. It commonly involves the skin, causing widespread itchy red patches.

ATLL is also likely to affect the **CNS** (the brain and spinal cord), especially if it **relapses**.

How is it treated?

Treatments for ATLL will vary from person to person because the nature of the lymphoma varies.

People with the most slowly growing types who feel generally well will probably be offered antiviral treatments. These help to fight the HTLV-1 virus and can slow the growth of certain forms of ATLL. The drugs used include alpha-interferon, zidovudine (Retrovir®), lamivudine (Epivir®), or zidovudine and lamivudine together (Combivir®).

If your lymphoma is growing more quickly and has more of the typical features of a lymphoma, you are likely to need chemotherapy too. The most common **regimen** is CHOP.

← You will find more information about CHOP chemotherapy on page 59.

Some people with ATLL who respond to chemotherapy will then be offered high-dose therapy and a stem cell transplant to reduce the risk of the lymphoma coming back.

Clinical trials continue to test new treatments for ATLL. You may be asked if you would like to take part in a clinical trial.

We produce a booklet on clinical trials. Please ring our helpline (0808 808 5555) or see our website (www.lymphomas.org.uk) if you would like a copy.

Nasal-type NK/T-cell lymphoma

What does it mean?
Nasal NK/T-cell lymphoma is a rare **extranodal** T-cell lymphoma. Extranodal means it grows outside of the lymphatic system, in this case in structures around the nose. Most of these lymphomas develop from 'natural killer' (NK) cells – another kind of **white blood cell**. A few develop from a **T cell**, so the name includes both.

Nasal lymphoma usually starts to grow in the sinuses. These are the air-filled spaces in the bones of your face that link to your nasal passages.

Who gets it?
This rare lymphoma occurs almost always in people from Asia and Central America.

It has been found that most people with nasal-type NK/T-cell lymphoma have had an infection with the Epstein–Barr virus (EBV) in the past. Exactly how the EBV infection is linked to this lymphoma is not yet clear.

How will it affect me?
Nasal lymphoma is most likely to be found only in the area around your nose. This means it is usually stage I or stage II lymphoma. You may hear it called stage IE or IIE – the 'E' stands for 'extranodal'.

The symptoms of nasal lymphoma usually affect the nose, eyes, mouth or face. You may have a blocked nose, discharge or bleeding from your nose, weepy eyes, swelling of your face, problems swallowing or dental problems.

High-grade non-Hodgkin lymphoma

In some people, the lymphoma is found in other parts of the body. For example, it can involve the bowel or cause a patchy rash on the skin.

How is it treated?
Nasal NK/T-cell lymphoma can be hard to treat successfully. It is usually treated with both chemotherapy and radiotherapy to the areas affected by the lymphoma.

Chemotherapy is used even if the lymphoma seems to be just within the nasal area. This is because the lymphoma often comes back in places outside the area treated with radiotherapy. Chemotherapy treats any lymphoma cells that might be lurking elsewhere but which cannot be seen.

The CHOP chemotherapy **regimen** may be used, but doctors often use other chemotherapy regimens to treat this lymphoma. These may include the drug L-asparaginase (Erwinase®). One regimen that seems to work well is known as SMILE – dexamethasone (a **s**teroid), **m**ethotrexate, **i**fosfamide, **L**-asparaginase and **e**toposide.

Non-Hodgkin lymphomas associated with immunodeficiency

Immunodeficiency means that the **immune system** is weakened. Someone with immunodeficiency is more prone to infections but they are also more likely to develop certain types of lymphoma.

Post-transplant lymphoproliferative disorder

What does it mean?
Post-transplant lymphoproliferative disorders (PTLDs) are a group of disorders that affect people who have had a transplant, such as a kidney, liver or bone marrow transplant.

Typically there is an increase (a 'proliferation') of certain **lymphocytes**. This is often linked to Epstein–Barr virus (EBV) infection. Some of these disorders turn into a type of high-grade non-Hodgkin lymphoma, most often a B-cell lymphoma.

Who gets it?
PTLDs develop in people taking **immunosuppressive** drugs that affect how well their **T cells** work. People taking these drugs after solid-organ transplants are 30–50 times more likely to develop non-Hodgkin lymphoma.

How will it affect me?
PTLD can cause of variety of symptoms. You may have one or more swollen **lymph nodes**. Some people also have other symptoms, such as weight loss, fever, night sweats and tiredness.

Extranodal lymphoma is quite common. For instance your bowel, lungs, liver or **CNS** (brain and spinal cord) may be affected. If you have had a solid-organ transplant, your transplanted organ may also be involved. At first, your doctors might suspect your symptoms are due to rejection of the organ.

How is it treated?
In some people, reducing or possibly stopping the immunosuppressive drugs can be enough to stop the abnormal cells growing. Stopping the drugs allows the T cells to start working again but this does mean you are more likely to reject your transplant. You will need to be carefully watched by your transplant doctors too. This approach is most likely to work if you have only recently had your transplant.

If this does not work or if it is some time since you had your transplant, you may be treated with the antibody rituximab. If you need stronger treatment, you may have rituximab together with chemotherapy, for example R-CHOP.

HIV-related lymphoma

What does it mean?
Lymphomas are more common in people who have something wrong with their **immune system**. This is the case for people who have **HIV** infection.

People with HIV are more likely to develop certain types of lymphoma. The most common ones are diffuse large B-cell lymphoma (DLBCL) and Burkitt lymphoma.

In the past, people with HIV were much more likely to have lymphoma in the brain and spinal cord – primary central nervous system lymphoma (PCNSL). With better treatment for HIV infection, this now happens less often.

Who gets it?
Anyone with HIV infection can develop lymphoma. The chances of getting non-Hodgkin lymphoma and the type of lymphoma will depend on how well the HIV is controlled.

With more use of good anti-retroviral treatment for HIV far fewer people now develop HIV-related lymphoma.

How will it affect me?
How your lymphoma affects you will depend on what kind of lymphoma you have. You will need to look at the information on your type of lymphoma elsewhere in this booklet. Your symptoms are likely to be much the same as they are in someone without HIV infection.

How is it treated?
What treatment you have will depend on what kind of lymphoma you have. The information on treatment in the section about your type of lymphoma will give you a guide. It is likely that you will be given the same treatment for your lymphoma as someone who does not have HIV infection.

Your risk of problems with infection will, however, be higher. This is because your immune system is already damaged and the treatment for your lymphoma will cause more damage.

High-grade non-Hodgkin lymphoma

Your HIV team will work closely with your lymphoma team. If you are taking anti-retroviral therapy, you should continue this when you are on chemotherapy. You should also continue to take any treatments you are already being given to avoid infections and keep you well, unless your doctors tell you to change.

The results of treating lymphoma in people being treated for HIV infection are now often very like those seen in people without HIV infection. You will, though, need extra care during your treatment to keep the chances of problems as low as possible.

Looking after yourself

Your feelings

Helping yourself

When someone close to you has lymphoma

6

Your feelings

No one can say exactly how you will feel when you learn you have high-grade lymphoma, when you are having treatment or afterwards. You will probably have all sorts of different feelings at different times. This is quite normal as there is no right or wrong way to handle things.

These are some of the feelings you may have:
- shock – you may feel numb and find it hard to accept things at first
- anxiety – you may be worried about your disease, your treatment, your future or your family
- sadness – your life and plans, at least for a time, are going to have to change
- fear – often this is fear of the unknown, so finding out more about what to expect can help
- anger – you may feel you've lost all control of your life and resent the fact that this has happened to you.

These feelings are all normal. It is important to accept them and give yourself time to deal with them. It's also important to talk about your feelings, especially if there are times when you are finding it harder to cope.

'It's all scary to begin with and you really do have to take one day at a time.'

Talking to someone close to you can sometimes be hard if they are dealing with their own feelings about your illness too. Your nurse specialist is often a good person to talk with or there may be specialist counsellors available at your hospital. Our helpline staff are ready to listen too (0808 808 5555). They may also be able to put you in touch with one of our 'buddies', who have all been affected by lymphoma too.

> 'The Lymphoma Association were always at the end of the line when I needed information or needed to talk to someone outside my family or circle of friends.'

Depression

You may feel that there are times when you don't want to talk and just want to be alone. This is quite normal but if you start to feel this all the time, it could be a sign of depression.

People who are depressed may also feel hopeless, guilty or worthless. They may have no interest in hobbies or normal activities and often find they wake very early or are sleeping all the time.

If you, or those around you, think you might be depressed, talk to someone about this. Depression will get worse if you don't do anything about it, but it can be successfully treated.

> 'There were many ups and downs. However, I've come through and am back at work. Hang in there – take each day as it comes, but look towards the time when it gets sorted.'

After treatment
Many people have very mixed feelings even when they have finished their treatment. Some people can feel more anxious and depressed at this stage, even if they have been told their treatment has been successful.

If this happens to you, it may be because you:
- start to think deeply about what has happened only once your treatment is finished
- are worried about the lymphoma coming back – you may get very anxious about further scans or check-ups and some people even start imagining symptoms at these times
- are still recovering from your treatment – sometimes side effects such as fatigue can last for months
- have had to make changes to your life because of the lymphoma or its treatment
- are worried about the future and find it hard to plan ahead.

> 'I had another scan and the results were very good – I was in remission! I expected to feel ecstatically happy but for a while I just felt scared that the cancer would come back.'

It is important to realise that these feelings are all normal, even if others expect you to feel happy. Talk to people, including your GP and hospital team, about how you are really feeling. Let them know too if you still have any side effects or symptoms. Our helpline staff and our 'buddies', who can understand how you are feeling, are also still there to listen when you have finished treatment (0808 808 5555).

Helping yourself

There are many things you can do to help yourself if you have non-Hodgkin lymphoma. These are a few suggestions.

Look after your general health and fitness
Many people find that having a serious illness makes them look again at their lifestyle. Changes that you make now may help you live a longer and healthier life after you have finished treatment.

It is important that you try to:
- drink plenty of liquids, especially if you are having chemotherapy
- eat a healthy diet – if you are having problems eating or are losing weight because of your treatment you should ask for advice about this first
- keep your body at a healthy weight
- stop smoking – lung infections are more common both with chemotherapy and with smoking; your risk of developing late side effects of treatment will also be higher if you smoke
- take regular exercise – research has shown that exercise can help reduce fatigue, as well as being good for your body generally.

'There are many things that trigger decisions in life; lymphoma was a major trigger for us. We now take each day as it comes and value each and every moment.'

You may want to look at other aspects of your life too, such as your responsibilities, your job or finances and how you spend your time. Many people find having lymphoma makes them value the simple things in life, such as spending time with family and friends and doing the activities they enjoy.

> You will find more information on looking after yourself, day-to-day life with lymphoma, your feelings and your relationships in our booklet *Living with lymphoma*. If you would like a copy please ring our helpline (0808 808 5555) or see our website (www.lymphomas.org.uk).

Find out about your lymphoma
Knowing more about your illness and your treatments can help in a number of ways, for example by:
- easing some of the fears and anxieties you may have
- picking up tips to avoid or reduce problems during and after treatment
- knowing how to deal with any side effects
- knowing when to call the hospital if a problem occurs
- helping you feel more in control of what is happening to you.

When someone close to you has lymphoma

When someone close to you has lymphoma it can be a hard time for you too. You may feel helpless watching the person you love going through all the tests and treatment. You may feel you don't know what to do or how to help.

Looking after yourself

There are lots of things you will be able to do, but don't forget to take care of yourself too. Make sure you look after your own health, particularly if you already have any illnesses, eat well and try to get plenty of rest. You will go through many of the same feelings as your loved one and will need time to deal with these too. Talk to someone if you are finding it hard to cope.

> 'Try to get some time for yourself, even if it is only fifteen minutes in the bath, time to go for a walk or just be alone in your room, whatever.'

People sometimes worry that they don't know what to say or will say the wrong thing. In fact, just being there, ready to listen, is often a huge help. Let the person know that you love and care for them, in whatever way you can – a smile or a hug may say much more than any words.

Practical things that may help your friend or loved one include:
- providing transport to hospital
- going along to hospital appointments with them to help remember what has been said
- helping with shopping or preparing meals
- taking care of other family members
- encouraging them to spend time seeing other people or doing something they enjoy
- organising fun things to do when they feel up to it.

➡ You might like to contact Carers UK, who can offer more free information, help and support. You will find their details on page 127.

Key facts

There is no right or wrong way to feel about having high-grade non-Hodgkin lymphoma. You will probably feel a mixture of shock, anxiety, sadness, fear and anger at different times.

If you or those around you think you may be depressed, talk to someone about this. Depression can be treated.

Finding out more about your illness and treatments can help you know what to expect and how to deal with problems. This can also help you feel more in control of what is happening to you.

Many people find having a serious illness makes them think about whether they need to change their lifestyle. Some changes could make you live a longer and healthier life after your treatment.

If someone close to you has lymphoma there are lots of practical things you can do to help, as well as ways to offer support. It is important though that you take care of yourself too and talk to someone if you are finding it hard to cope.

Help and support

Whatever your situation is, we hope that this booklet has helped you to understand more about high-grade non-Hodgkin lymphoma, particularly the type that is most relevant to you, and the sort of treatments your doctors are likely to recommend.

If you would like further information about anything mentioned in this booklet, or would like to talk to someone, please get in touch with us.

How we can help

Helpline – The Lymphoma Association helpline is there to offer a listening ear for you, your family and friends. Your call will be confidential and free. Please ring us on 0808 808 5555 if you would like to talk about any aspect of lymphoma or about how you are feeling. Our helpline is open from Monday to Friday (please see our website for the current opening hours). You can also email the helpline on information@lymphomas.org.uk or contact them via Live Chat on our website.

Lymphoma Association buddy scheme – Many people feel more encouraged and supported after speaking to other people affected by lymphoma. Even if their experience was not exactly the same as yours, it can be a relief to speak with someone who has been through something similar. We may be able to put you in touch by telephone or email with one of our buddies.

Help and support

Lymphoma Association support groups – There are support groups for people with lymphoma around the UK. Please ring our helpline for more information or use the 'search' facility on our website to find your nearest group.

Online – We have forums on our website where you can share what has happened to you. We are also on Facebook, Twitter and YouTube.

Lymphoma matters – You can subscribe to our free quarterly magazine, which is full of up-to-date information about lymphoma, reports on the latest research and new treatments, articles on living with lymphoma and interviews with people affected by lymphoma.

Free information – We have lots of information on lymphoma and its treatment on our website (www.lymphomas.org.uk). We also produce a series of booklets about lymphoma. These can be downloaded or ordered from our website and are all free of charge. You can also ask for booklets to be sent to you by ringing our helpline on 0808 808 5555 or by email (information@lymphomas.org.uk).

How you can help us

We continually strive to improve our information resources for people affected by lymphoma and we would be interested in any feedback you might have on this booklet. Please visit www.lymphomas.org.uk/feedback or email publications@lymphomas.org.uk if you have any comments. Or if you prefer, please ring our helpline on 0808 808 5555.

Glossary

Allogeneic the use of someone else's tissue (eg stem cells)

Anaemia lack of red blood cells in the blood, often talked about as the level of haemoglobin

Anaesthetic drugs given to make a part of the body numb (a local anaesthetic) or put the whole body to sleep (a general anaesthetic)

Antibody a protein that sticks to disease-causing cells or organisms, such as bacteria, leading to their death

Autologous the use of a person's own tissue (eg stem cells)

B cell the same as a B lymphocyte, a white blood cell that normally helps to fight infections by making antibodies

Bacteria small organisms, some of which can cause infections and disease

Biopsy a test that takes some cells to be looked at under a microscope

Blood count a blood test that counts the cells in your blood, including the red blood cells, the different kinds of white blood cells, and platelets

Glossary

Bone marrow — spongy material at the centre of our bones; produces the body's blood cells

CNS — central nervous system, the name for the brain and spinal cord together

Cycle — a block of chemotherapy that is followed by a rest period to allow the normal healthy cells to recover

Diagnosis — deciding what an illness or disease is; giving it a name

Diaphragm — a sheet of muscle that separates the chest from the abdomen (see picture on page 10)

Extranodal — refers to a lymphoma that forms in an area outside of the lymphatic system, for example in the gut or bone marrow

Haematologist — a doctor who specialises in diseases of the blood and blood cells

HIV — human immunodeficiency virus, a virus that causes weakness in part of the immune system leading to AIDS (acquired immune deficiency syndrome)

Immune system — the parts of the body that fight off and prevent infection

Immuno-deficiency — weakness in or a breakdown of a person's ability to fight infections

Immuno-suppressive — prevents the immune system working as it normally would

Intravenous — into a vein

Glossary

Lymphocyte	a type of white blood cell that normally helps to fight infections; may be either a B lymphocyte or a T lymphocyte
Lymph node	gland acting like a sieve in the lymphatic system; involved in fighting infection
Neutropenia	a lack of neutrophils in the blood, which makes you prone to infection
Neutrophil	a type of white blood cell that is important in fighting infections caused by bacteria or fungus
Oncologist	a doctor who specialises in treating cancer
Pathologist	a doctor who looks at and tests diseased tissues to make a diagnosis
Platelets	the tiny fragments of cells in your blood that help form blood clots and stop bleeding
Prophylaxis	a treatment given to prevent an illness or problem developing in the future
Protein	matter found in living things with many roles, including helping to control how our cells work and fighting infections
Radiographer	a person who takes X-rays or gives radiotherapy
Radiologist	a doctor who can analyse X-rays and scans
Radiotherapist	a doctor who specialises in radiotherapy (also often known as a clinical oncologist)

Glossary

Red blood cell   a cell that contains the red pigment haemoglobin, which allows it to carry oxygen around the body

Refractory   meaning an illness that has not responded well to treatment

Regimen   a combination of drugs given together in a set pattern

Relapse   to come back after treatment

Spleen   a organ about the size of a closed fist behind the stomach that is part of the immune system

Splenomegaly   a term meaning that the spleen is larger than normal

Subcutaneous   underneath the skin

Symptom   something you notice or feel when you have an illness

T cell   the same as a T lymphocyte, a white blood cell that normally helps to fight infections caused by viruses

Thrombo-cytopenia   a lack of platelets in the blood, which makes you more prone to bleeding or bruising

Virus   tiny organisms, some of which can cause infection and disease

White blood cell   a cell found in the blood and in many other tissues that helps our bodies to fight infections; there are several different kinds including lymphocytes and neutrophils

Useful organisations

This is a short list of useful organisations, but there are many others. If you can't find the right organisation listed here, please ring our helpline (0808 808 5555).

British Association for Counselling and Psychotherapy
Has a register of accredited counsellors throughout the UK.
 01455 883300
www.bacp.co.uk
 bacp@bacp.co.uk

Cancer Research UK
Offers information and statistics on all kinds of cancer, including treatment, prevention, screening and research. A team of specialist cancer nurses can be contacted by phone by calling their Freephone number.
 0808 800 4040 (Monday–Friday, 9am–5pm)
www.cancerhelp.org.uk
 via website

Carers UK
Offers free and confidential information for carers.
 0808 808 7777
www.carersuk.org
 via website

Infertility Network UK
Gives information and emotional support to those affected by infertility
 0800 008 7464 (Monday–Thursday, 9am–4pm)
www.infertilitynetworkuk.com
 via website

Useful organisations

Leukaemia & Lymphoma Research

Funds research into the causes and treatment of leukaemia, lymphoma and related diseases.

📞 020 7504 2200 (Monday–Friday, 9am–5pm)

www.leukaemialymphomaresearch.org.uk

✉ info@beatingbloodcancers.org.uk

Macmillan Cancer Support

Offers practical, medical, emotional and financial support to people living with cancer.

📞 0808 808 0000 (Monday–Friday, 9am–8pm)

www.macmillan.org.uk

✉ via website

Maggie's Cancer Caring Centres

Offers a network of drop-in centres throughout the UK (as well as an 'online' centre) with the aim of supporting people with cancer, their family and friends.

📞 0300 123 1801

www.maggiescentres.org

✉ enquiries@maggiescentres.org

Selected references

The full list of references is available on request. Please contact us via email (publications@lymphomas.org.uk) or telephone 01296 619409 if you would like a copy.

Books
Swerdlow SH, et al (eds). *WHO Classification of Tumours of Haematopoietic and Lymphoid Tissues.* 2008. IARC, Lyon.

Hatton C, et al. *Lymphoma.* 2008. Health Press: Oxford.

Journal articles
McMillan A, et al. Guideline on the prevention of secondary central nervous system lymphoma: *British Committee for Standards in Haematology.* British Journal of Haematology, 2013. 163: 168–181.

Shustov A. Novel therapies for peripheral T-cell lymphomas. *Therapeutic Advances in Hematology*, 2013. 4: 173–187.

Dunleavy K, Wilson WH. How I treat HIV-associated lymphoma. *Blood*, 2012. 119: 3245–3255.

Cultrera JL, Dalia SM. Diffuse large B-cell lymphoma: current strategies and future directions. *Cancer Control*, 2012. 19: 204–213.

Federico M, et al. Clinicopathologic characteristics of angioimmunoblastic T-cell lymphoma: analysis of the International Peripheral T-Cell Lymphoma Project. *Journal of Clinical Oncology*, 2012. 31: 240-246.

McKay P, et al. Guidelines for the investigation and management of mantle cell lymphoma. *British Journal of Haematology*, 2012. 159: 405–426.

Other sources
Cancer Research UK. *UK cancer incidence statistics 2011.* Available at: www.cancerresearchuk.org/cancer-info/cancerstats/types/nhl (accessed June 2014).

Appendix: Tips for coping with treatment side effects

The following information suggests possible ways of dealing with side effects. This is only introductory information – be sure to ask your medical team for advice about dealing with your side effects.

Generally speaking you should tell your team if you feel unwell in any way.

For more information about dealing with specific side effects please call us on 0808 808 5555.

Low white cell count (neutropenia)

Call the hospital **at once** if you develop signs of infection such as fever, temperature of 38°C or above, or chills, shivering or sweating.

⬅ Other possible signs of infection are listed on page 50.

The following tips may help you lower your risk of developing an infection:

Wash well and regularly. Wash hands before meals, after using the toilet, after using public facilities.

Avoid places where infection risk is increased, such as swimming pools, crowded shops and buses.

Avoid contact with people who have infections (including chickenpox).

Appendix: Tips for coping with treatment side effects

Don't eat anything that is past its sell-by date and eat refrigerated food within 24 hours once it has been opened.

Avoid foods that contain lots of live **bacteria**. These include:

- unpasteurised cheeses
- takeaways
- raw or undercooked eggs
- live or probiotic yoghurt (pasteurised yoghurt is fine)
- peppercorns
- undercooked meats and fish
- pâté.

Ask your nurse for information on 'clean' or 'safe' diets.

Take care when handling pets – avoid bites or scratches and wash your hands afterwards. If possible, ask someone else to deal with litter trays and pet faeces.

Wear gloves for gardening.

Low red cell count (anaemia)

Tell your doctor if you feel short of breath, abnormally tired or have abnormal aches and pains.

Ask about what treatment you could have for anaemia.

Low platelet count (thrombocytopenia)

Tell your hospital team about bruising or bleeding. Call the hospital at once if you feel very unwell, faint or clammy.

Avoid contact sports or very vigorous exercise.

Take care to avoid injury when doing day-to-day things like cooking and gardening.

Appendix: Tips for coping with treatment side effects

Feeling sick

Take anti-sickness drugs.

Tell one of your hospital team if they don't work.

Try travel sickness wristbands from the pharmacy. These prevent nausea by using acupressure points.

Try relaxation techniques.

Avoid cooking smells and seek help with preparing meals.

Eat smaller meals that are cold or at room temperature.

Keep your surroundings as peaceful and clean as possible, and try to get some fresh air.

Change in taste and loss of appetite

Try to eat little and often and avoid big meals. Eat whenever you are hungry, whether or not this is your usual mealtime.

Try foods that taste stronger – marinated foods, savoury rather than sweet. Eat food warm rather than hot.

Rinse your mouth before meals and follow any mouth-care regimen you've been given.

Have a ready supply of things that are quick and easy to prepare.

Try to supplement your diet with nutritious drinks, but not at mealtimes. Drinking through a straw may be helpful.

Eat with others in a pleasant environment.

Take gentle exercise when possible.

Appendix: Tips for coping with treatment side effects

Constipation

Ask your doctor if your treatment might cause constipation and ask about using laxatives to prevent it.

Make sure you drink plenty and eat a high-fibre diet.

Try a hot drink in the mornings. Take gentle exercise when possible.

Diarrhoea

Tell you hospital team if you are having several episodes of diarrhoea a day, if it continues for more than 24 hours or if you have any abdominal pain.

Ensure you have an adequate fluid intake.

Sore mouth

Visit your dentist before starting treatment and tell a member of your hospital team if you need dental work during your treatment.

Avoid smoking and drinking alcohol as these can make any soreness worse.

Practise good oral hygiene – the hospital may prescribe special mouthwashes for you to use. Avoid mouthwashes containing salt or alcohol.

Use a soft-bristled toothbrush and rinse your mouth after meals. Keep your lips moist with lip creams or Vaseline™.

Avoid hot, spicy foods or foods that are coarse in texture. Cool, easy-to-swallow things can help, such as ice cream and yoghurt. Sip drinks through a straw.

Speak to your hospital team about taking painkillers.

Appendix: Tips for coping with treatment side effects

Fatigue

Take regular light exercise, such as walking.

Take regular short rests throughout the day.

Ask your doctor if you are anaemic, and whether any treatment will help your anaemia.

Ask if any of your medicines cause fatigue and if these can be changed or stopped.

Plan your activities: do a bit less of what's less important, and plan important things for when you have more energy.

Accept offers of help with day-to-day tasks.

Aim to get a good night's sleep.

Eat as well as possible.

Make time to see friends and take part in normal social activities.

Hair loss

Have your hair cut short before you start treatment.

Wearing a hairnet or towelling turban to bed will help to collect hair lost overnight.

Talk about wigs with your hospital team, or try hats or scarves.

Use wide-toothed combs and soft-bristled hairbrushes.

Avoid things that pull at your hair such as hair straighteners, rollers and tight elastics. Avoid using heated rollers or hairdryers.

Avoid chemical treatments such as perms and hair dyes. This also applies when your hair first starts to grow back as results can be unpredictable; you might want to try vegetable-based dyes at first.

Protect your head from sun and wind to stop the skin of your scalp becoming dry.

Use make-up, jewellery and accessories to give you more confidence.

Peripheral neuropathy

Tell your doctors or nurses if you have pins and needles or loss of feeling in your fingers or toes, loss of balance, abdominal pain or constipation.

Take care to avoid injury to your fingers and toes, which will be less sensitive than usual: avoid extreme temperatures, wear gloves for gardening and take care when cooking.

Keep your feet and hands warm as cold can make symptoms worse.

Try gentle massage and exercise your fingers and toes by flexing and stretching them for a few minutes four times a day.

Wear comfortable shoes – avoid high heels or shoes that are tight.

Check your feet regularly for damaged skin in parts that are numb, particularly on the soles of your feet and around your toenails.

Sore skin

Ask your team for advice about looking after your skin.

Do not use creams unless recommended by your doctor. Avoid soaps, talcum powder and deodorants.

Avoid rubbing the skin. If bathing, use lukewarm water and pat dry with a towel.

Use electric razors rather than wet shaving.

Protect your skin from sun and wind.